PREDICTIVE MEDICINE

PREDICTIVE MEDICINE

A Study in Strategy...

E. Cheraskin, M.D., D.M.D.
W. M. Ringsdorf, Jr., D.M.D.

82   7335-2

Keats Publishing, Inc.
New Canaan, Connecticut

**Your only insurance
against tomorrow is
what you do today!**
Sir William Osler

Contents

Preface

Goethe said it succinctly: "Everything has been thought of before, but the difficulty is to think of it again." It will therefore not come as a surprise that there is likely nothing new in this monograph. As a matter of fact, the overriding importance of health as against illness was known to the Chinese eons ago. Their writings reveal that they compensated the physician while well and the contract was clear that the compensation was for staying well. Illness became expensive, not in economic terms, but in pain, incapacitation, grief, and death. Sickness was also costly to the physician because he had already been compensated for the preservation of health.

Today there are still disciples in the field of health-maintenance. However, they are few and far between and work with limited funds and facilities in, more or less, cloisters. But these researchers have learned the Chinese lesson well and have refined the ancient techniques in the light of present-day technology.

Hence, all that is unprecedented about this monograph is simply that it attempts to paint a picture, necessarily in broad strokes, of the anatomy of a health program. It is the dream of the authors that what lies within these pages will serve as a *stroma* for a predictive medicine system. It is our earnest hope that others, more knowledgeable, will contribute the *parenchyma*. In any case, the time is ripe to reinstate the old Chinese system; and, possibly, this monograph will serve as a catalyst for such a movement.

E. Cheraskin, M.D., D.M.D.
W. M. Ringsdorf, Jr., D.M.D., M.S.

Acknowledgements

There are many to whom we are beholden. Certainly, the scores of investigators who generated the fundamental research which led to the birth of this book must be applauded. Our heartfelt thanks go to our secretaries, Mrs. Alda McDowell, Mrs. Clara Benton, and Mrs. Edna Bronson, for their patience with countless behind-the-scenes duties. Our appreciation to Mrs. Sarah Brown and her library staff for their cooperation in our seemingly endless literature searches. Our gratitude to the administration of the University of Alabama in Birmingham Medical Center for creating the environment without which this monograph would not have been possible. Finally, feedback from some of the material in this book was possible because of cooperation given us by the *Alabama Journal of Medical Sciences* and the *Journal of the American Geriatrics Society,* where sections had been earlier published.

E. Cheraskin, M.D., D.M.D.
W. M. Ringsdorf, Jr., D.M.D., M.S.

Definitions

The manner in which man is to exercise his instrumentality for the prevention of disease, the prevention of the vestiges of disease, and the prevention of fatality in disease, is to search out those earliest evasive periods of defect in the physiological state, and to adopt measures for their remedy. This appears to me to be highest, the most ennobled duty of the physician, calling for the most abstruse knowledge of the science of life, the deepest experience in disease, the keenest exercise of the perceptive faculties, the calmest, most farsighted reasoning, and the wisest judgment—a duty as much above the management of acute disease as to rule an empire is above fighting a pitched battle.   —Dobell.

For pragmatic purposes and as an immediate working hypothesis, *predictive medicine* may be defined as the clinical discipline designed to *anticipate* disease in man.[1] The intent, by such an approach, is to *foretell* illness before it erupts in its classical form. This postulate will be considered in detail in chapter 4. Predictive medicine emphasizes *primary* prevention (prevention of occurrence). Such a philosophy immediately delineates *predictive medicine* from *conventional medicine* where the cardinal theme, by act if not by word, is the *identification* of existing disease with subsequent treatment and, at best, *secondary* prevention (prevention of recurrence).

Historical Considerations

Predictive medicine is not new.[2] Hippocrates recognized that in the female there was a striking positive parallelism between obesity, menstrual aberrations, and sterility. Since that time and up to the present, scores of publications have sought to underline the prognosticative worth of many and diverse clinical, biochemical, social, psychologic, and economic parameters with regard to different disease states.

All of these studies possess one common denominator.

1

Namely, they all seek variables *within* man to explain why he succumbs to illness. A rumination of the historical course of *health concepts* brings this point into sharp focus.

Before the Germ Theory. In the beginning, health and disease were acknowledged to be God-given. When man sinned, he was cursed with ill health. When he behaved, he went unscathed. The dogma was understandable, since life and death, even in those early times, was so inextricably linked with religion.

However, the explanation for the causes for health and disease slowly changed. Increasingly, more attention was directed *within* man as the root of problems. In other words, the body was viewed as the *soil* in which disease flourished. While many of the ancient theories have now been discredited, the denominator which has persisted, even to this day, is that the *internal milieu* of man is inextricably associated with the medical problems which beset him.

The Germ Theory. For approximately twenty-five hundred years medicine has been probing for the roots of illness. Until the advent of microbiology, as we have just learned, disease was ascribed to a turbulence in man's inner world. Then came Pasteur and his colleagues and the birth of the germ theory. This relatively simple hypothesis suggested that germs are *seeds* which, when implanted, beget disease. The proposition, like any new concept, had its difficulties in acceptance. But it won because it was simple, convincing, and most important, comfortable. Now man could blame the cosmos and so regard his infirmities as part of his uncontrolled destiny.

Beyond the Germ Theory. There is no question but that microbes are *involved* in many illnesses. However, microbial participation does not argue that the microorganism is the mainspring. Moreover, the germ theory does not resolve the many contradictions which are so frequently encountered in nature. Why, for example, can two seemingly similar souls breathe the very same viruses at precisely the same time and yet only one "catches a cold"? Hence, there are penetrating and perturbing paradoxes in the field of so-called microbial disease where it is abundantly clear that microorganisms are *involved* and thought to be the simple *cause.* But, even more importantly, how does one unravel the rising and insolvable problems of chronic disease where microbiology plays less of a role? What are the causes of arteriosclerosis, cancer, rheumatoid arthritis, glaucoma, and multiple sclerosis?

These and many other enigmas now have brought science to a thesis of health and disease *beyond* the germ hypothesis. As a matter of fact, the current interpretation of the genesis of health and disease is a marriage of the before-the-germ-theory *and* the germ-theory. It recognizes that disease, for practical purposes gauged by clinical symptoms and signs, is the end-result of an environmental challenge. The peripheral threat, the seed, may be microbial; but it is also likely to be physical, chemical, or psychic. In this connection, the new philosophy concedes the importance of the external milieu but enlarges upon the scope of the challenges. For instance, there is a rising interest in pollution as a pathogenic factor. But, at the same time, the modern theories of illness appreciate the fact that the capacity of man to withstand the external bombardment is an equally vital ingredient. This latter element is cloaked in such terms as *host resistance, host susceptibility, tissue tolerance, constitution, predisposition,* or *proneness.* The whole topic of host state will receive more detailed attention in chapter 3.

The name of Pasteur is inextricably linked with the germ hypothesis. What is not generally appreciated is that Pasteur also recognized the cardinal role of host resistance and susceptibility. Repeatedly, Pasteur and his colleagues expressed the conviction that the *terrain,* as he chose to call it, of the infected body often determines the course of the infectious process. In one sense, he anticipated the statement by George Bernard Shaw that the characteristic microbe of a disease is more likely to be a symptom and not the cause of the problem.

The New Terminology

Thus, as we have learned, predictive medicine is not new.[3-27] It is cloaked under diverse terms such as *preventative, prognostic, protective, anticipatory, social medicine,* and *propetology.* All of these labels are perfectly respectable, descriptive, valid, and useful. One might then question the need for generating new nomenclature such as *predictive medicine.* Four explanations are offered. First, from a purely etymologic standpoint, *predictive medicine* is the most precise term, since the Latin derivative for prediction means to foretell. Hence, the term *predictive medicine* spells out unequivocally the unique anticipatory characteristic of this philosophy of medicine. Second, unlike the apt term *propetology* which means "leaning toward," *predictive medicine* is a simple and self-explanatory term. Third, *predictive medicine,* as a relatively new label, is not shrouded with historic misconceptions and semantic overtones. For example, present-day preventative medicine is largely concerned with public health in the traditional sense (acute infectious diseases) and embraces relatively few prognostic connotations relating to the common chronic killing and crippling disorders (e.g., ischemic heart disease, cancer, rheumatoid arthritis). Fourth, *predictive medicine* is a unique discipline which encompasses concepts and instrumentation from many different well-established specialties (e.g., epidemiology, biostatistics, clinical pathology, clinical medicine, psychology, ecology, nutrition, physical education, and stomatology) which are not currently utilized in *packaged form* in any other single discipline.

Health Versus Disease Detection

There are presently in operation over two hundred *alleged* health programs.[25] A number of examples come to mind to underline the basic distinction between the fundamentals of

4

predictive medicine versus existing *health evaluation systems.* For instance, there is no question regarding the desirability of a periodic vaginal Papanicolaou smear for the detection of gynecologic cancer. The hope, always, is that the smear will prove to be negative. Obviously, this testing technique is to be applauded, and women should be encouraged to undergo this periodic checkup. In the event that the results are negative, the patient is requested to return at a later date (usually in six to twelve months depending upon age) for another *health* checkup, as it is usually phrased. There is no question but that periodic reexamination is desirable. At each revisit the hope prevails, by both the patient and the doctor, that the smear will continue to prove negative. This is also admittedly a commendable goal. Unfortunately, sooner or later, the smear may be positive. Hence, it becomes necessary in the present traditional medicine to institute surgery and/or irradiation. This, again, is desirable since all will concur that *early* detection and treatment prove more successful and yield a better prognosis than cancer recognition and therapy in later stages.

There is, in the sequence just outlined, one serious semantic trap with significant practical overtones. While all that has been described is to be applauded as a demonstration of therapeutic medicine, the one point overlooked is that the procedure is *not* a *health examination* but rather a *disease detection* program.

Ideally, a *true* health examination commences with a patient's showing a negative smear. Additionally, this evaluation should allow the opportunity to point out to the patient her degree of cancer proneness. Finally, a true health appraisal should include proper counsel so that the patient is provided with whatever information is available to *reduce* the risk of cancer (see chapter 2). Hence, it is obvious that the traditional *health* examination is, in fact, a *disease* detection program. There is a justifiable niche for such a system in present-day medicine. However, there is also a crying need for a *true health evaluation and maintenance program.*[28-29] This, in simple terms, is the purpose of this monograph.

Summary

Since the time of Hippocrates it has been known that different types of people display different illnesses. More recently information has been compiled to indicate that there are disparate sorts of individuals. Now medicine is beginning to learn to identify the diverse kinds of maladies which beset different kinds of people. Hence, there is a developing body of facts which makes it possible to *anticipate* disease. The chapter to follow will underscore this point with a demonstration of one already available experimental model and another in a more embryonic form.

References

1. Cheraskin, E. and Ringsdorf, W. M., Jr. *Predictive medicine: I. Definitions.* Alabama J. Med. Sci. 7:4, 444-447, October 1970.

2. Draper, G., Dupertuis, C. W., and Caughey, J. L., Jr. *Human constitution in clinical medicine.* 1944. New York, Paul B. Hoeber.

3. Cheraskin, E. and Ringsdorf, W. M., Jr. *The health of the dentist and his wife: a predictive health program.* J. South. California Dent. Assn. 37:7, 271-276, July 1969.

4. Cheraskin, E. and Ringsdorf, W. M., Jr. *The health of the dentist and his wife: present findings in a predictive health program.* J. South. California Dent. Assn. 37:9, 413-421, September 1969.

5. Cheraskin, E., Ringsdorf, W. M., Jr., and Aspray, D. W. *Cancer proneness profile: a study in ponderal index and blood glucose.* Geriatrics 24:8, 121-125, August 1969.

6. Cheraskin, E., Ringsdorf, W. M., Jr., Setyaadmadja, A. T. S. H., Barrett, R. A., Aspray, D. W., and Curry, S. *Cancer proneness profile: a study in weight and blood glucose.* Geriatrics 23:4, 134-137, April 1968.

7. Cheraskin, E., Ringsdorf, W. M., Jr., Setyaadmadja, A. T. S. H., Barrett, R. A., Sibley, G. T., and Reid, R. W. *Environmental factors in blood glucose regulation.* J. Amer. Geriat. Soc. 16:7, 823-825, July 1968.

8. Cheraskin, E., Ringsdorf, W. M., Jr., Setyaadmadja, A. T. S. H., and Barrett, R. A. *Biochemical profile in predictive medicine.* In Poyer, J., Herrick, J., and Weber, T. B. *Biomedical sciences instrumentation.* 1967. Pittsburgh, Instrument Society of America. pp. 3-15.

9. Cheraskin, E., Ringsdorf, W. M., Jr., Setyaadmadja, A. T. S. H., and Barrett, R. A. *Clinical chemistry and predictive medicine.* J. Med. Assn. St. Alabama 36:11, 1337-1340, May 1967.

10. Cheraskin, E., Ringsdorf, W. M., Jr., Setyaadmadja, A. T. S. H., and Barrett, R. A. *Coronary proneness and carbohydrate metabolism: glucose effect on dextrinization time.* Geriatrics 22:9, 122-126, September 1967.

11. Cheraskin, E., Ringsdorf, W. M., Jr., Setyaadmadja, A. T. S. H., and Barrett, R. A. *Predictive dentistry: the Cornell Medical Index Health Questionnaire [general responses] and dental findings.* New York J. Dent. 37:3, 104-107, March 1967.

12. Dorn, H. F. *Tobacco consumption and mortality from cancer and other diseases.* Pub. Health Rep. 74:7, 581-585, July 1959.

13. Galdston, I. *The meaning of social medicine.* 1954. Cambridge, Harvard University Press.

14. Levy, R. L., White, P. D., Stroud, W. P., and Hillman, C. C. *Overweight: its prognostic significance.* J. A. M. A. 131:12, 951-953, July 1946.

15. Marks, H. H. *Influence of obesity on morbidity and mortality.* Bull. New York Acad. Med. 36:4, 296-312, May 1960.

16. Sadusk, J. F. and Robbins, L. C. *Proposal for health-hazard appraisal in comprehensive health care.* J. A. M. A. 203:13, 1108-1112, 25 March 1968.

17. Setyaadmadja, A. T. S. H., Cheraskin, E., Ringsdorf, W. M., Jr., and Barrett, R. A. *Predictive prosthodontics. I. General health status and edentulousness.* J. Prosthet. Dent. 21:5, 475-479, May 1969.

18. Symposium: *Measuring the risk of coronary heart disease in adult population groups.* Amer. J. Pub. Health 47: Suppl. 4, April 1957.

19. Ungerleider, H. E. *The prognostic implications of the electrocardiogram.* In Higgins, E. V., Jecklin, H., Tanner, E., and Ungerleider, H. E. *Annals of life insurance medicine.* Berlin, Summer 1962.

20. Vecchio, T. J. *Predictive value of a single diagnostic test in unselected populations.* New England J. Med. 274:21, 1171-1173, 26 May 1966.

21. Williams, R. J. and Siegel, F. L. *Editorial: "Propetology," a new branch of medical science.* Amer. J. Med. 31:3, 325-327, September 1961.

22. Epstein, F. H. *Predicting coronary heart disease.* J. A. M. A. 201:11, 795-800, 11 September 1967.

23. Thorner, R. M. *Whither multiphasic screening?* New England J. Med. 280:19, 1037-1042, 8 May 1969.

24. Still, J. W. *Adult preventive medicine: the fourth phase in the evolution of medicine.* J. Amer. Geriat. Soc. 16:4, 395-406, April 1968.

25. Schoen, A. W. *Automated multiphasic health testing programs directory,* 1971-1972, second edition. Burbank, Bioscience Publications, Inc.

26. Gelman, A. C. *Automated multiphasic health testing.* Pub. Health Rep. 85:4, 361-373, April 1970.

27. Schuman, L. M. *Approaches to primary prevention of disease.* Pub. Health Rep. 85:1, 1-10, January 1970.

28. Marxer, W. L. and Cowgill, G. R. *The art of predictive medicine.* 1967. Springfield, Charles C. Thomas.

29. Robbins, L. C. and Hall, J. H. *How to practice prospective medicine.* 1970. Indianapolis, Methodist Hospital of Indiana.

7

Experimental Models

There is a very ancient belief that health is a simple state to be obtained by observing a few simple positive and negative rules. . . . But it follows from the complexity of the body that health cannot be a simple state. . . . Because there are literally thousands of ways of becoming ill, to be well, one has to be well in thousands of ways at once.   —Sir Russell Brain.

In chapter 1, consideration was given to the definition of *predictive medicine.* Cursory circumspection was accorded the unique attributes of such a philosophy in the health sciences. An illustration was offered to underline the fundamental delineation between an *alleged* health program, in reality a disease-detection evaluation, versus a *true* predictive health system as it should prevail in the case of gynecologic cancer. Proneness profiles, designed to *anticipate* rather than to *identify* disease, are now being developed. A discussion of two such experimental models will be the theme of this chapter.[1] One, the *coronary proneness profile,* has been extensively studied and now allows great predictive potential. The other, a *cancer proneness profile,* is much more recent and has been less investigated. Since it is still in the process of development, its predictive worth is limited.

Coronary Proneness Profile

It is abundantly evident that coronary artery disease is epidemic today in the United States.[2] For example, the possibility of a heart attack in presumably healthy male subjects before the age of sixty is about 20 percent. The need for primary prevention (prevention of occurrence), as indicated in chapter 1, is heightened by the facts that (1) acute mortality approaches 40 percent, and (2) half of this latter group, or about 20 percent of first attacks, terminate in death within 60 minutes after the initial symptoms and signs appear. Clearly, it is imperative to perfect and activate a *primary* prevention treatment program. Such a profile is a function of a number of already-identified parameters including (1) age and sex, (2) serum lipids, (3) blood pressure, (4) weight, (5) blood glucose, (6) uric acid, (7) diet, (8) tobacco consumption, (9) physical activity, (10) electrocardiography, (11) family history, and (12) personality structure.

Age and Sex. It will be learned that age is a highly significant parameter in predictive systems (chapters 4, 5, and

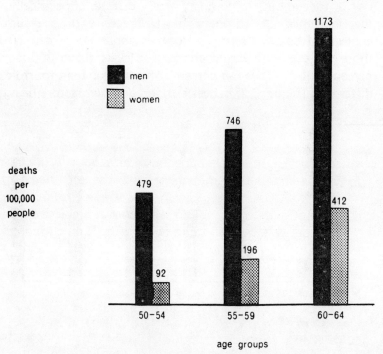

Keys, A. The individual risk of coronary artery disease.
Ann. New York Acad. Sc. 134:#2, 1046–1056, 28 February 1966.

Figure 2-1. The death rate ascribed to arteriosclerotic heart disease according to age and sex.

8-15). A number of studies in many countries have unveiled the mortality rates ascribed to atherosclerotic heart disease. Two features are most prominent. First, the death rate rises with advancing age. Second, the patterns in the sexes are vastly different. For example, the deaths in 1960 per 100,000 men and women in the United States are pictured in figure 2-1. *Thus, the evidence indicates that age and maleness must be viewed as major coronary risk factors.*[3]

Serum Lipids. The overall predictive potential of serum cholesterol will be analyzed later (chapters 5, 6, 8, 9). It is now quite clear that the higher the serum cholesterol concentration in an allegedly healthy man, the greater is his risk of succumbing to coronary artery disease.[4] Specifically, the incidence of coronary heart disease with a serum cholesterol below 200 mg. percent is about 1.5 percent. In those subjects with serum cholesterol levels above 300 mg. percent, the figure is 6.5 percent. This greater than fourfold difference (figure 2-2) suggests that, all other factors being

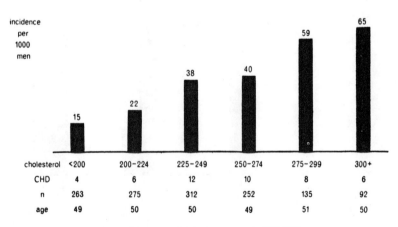

incidence per 1000 men					
cholesterol	<200	200–224	225–249	250–274	275–299	300+
CHD	4	6	12	10	8	6
n	263	275	312	252	135	92
age	49	50	50	49	51	50

People's Gas, Light, and Coke Company study, 1958-1962.

Figure 2-2. The relationship of serum cholesterol and the subsequent incidence of new clinical coronary heart disease.

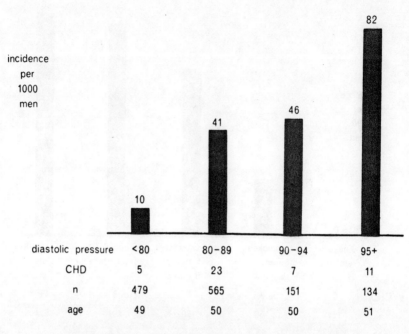

diastolic pressure	<80	80-89	90-94	95+
CHD	5	23	7	11
n	479	565	151	134
age	49	50	50	51

People's Gas, Light, and Coke Company study, 1958-1962.

Figure 2-3. The relationship of diastolic blood pressure and the subsequent incidence of new clinical coronary heart disease.

equal, *elevated serum cholesterol is a major coronary risk factor.*

Blood Pressure. It is noteworthy that the incidence of coronary artery disease is approximately 1 percent in subjects with diastolic pressure under 80 mm. Hg (figure 2-3). In contrast, the incidence is 8.2 percent with diastolic pressure greater than 95 mm. Hg. The intermediate blood pressure groups are paralleled by intermediate risk. *It is, therefore, clear that, all other factors constant, hypertension may be viewed as a major coronary risk factor.*[5]

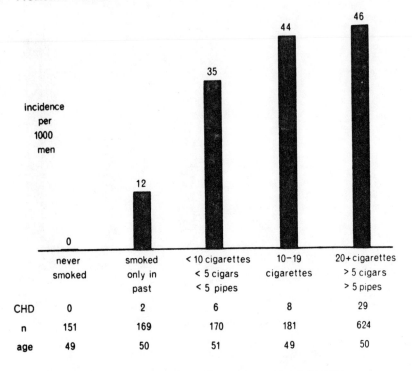

	never smoked	smoked only in past	< 10 cigarettes < 5 cigars < 5 pipes	10–19 cigarettes	20+ cigarettes > 5 cigars > 5 pipes
CHD	0	2	6	8	29
n	151	169	170	181	624
age	49	50	51	49	50

People's Gas, Light, and Coke Company study, 1958-1962.

Figure 2-4. The incidence of clinical coronary heart disease in terms of tobacco consumption.

Tobacco Consumption. For practical purposes, with regard to tobacco intake, cigarette smoking is the prime risk factor when weighed against pipe and cigar usage. The evidence indicates that the ex-smoker shows an incidence of 1.2 percent coronary artery disease (figure 2-4). In the individual consuming less than ten cigarettes daily, the incidence climbs almost threefold to 3.5 percent. With 10 to 19 cigarettes and 20 or more per day, the figures reach 4.4 and 4.6 percent, respectively. *Hence, all other variables being constant, cigarette consumption must be considered as a major coronary risk factor.*[6]

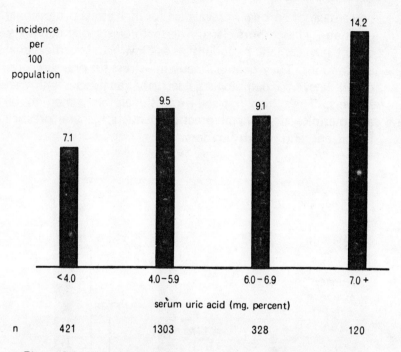

Figure 2-5. The incidence of coronary heart disease in terms of serum uric acid concentration.

Other Single Risk Variables. Mention was made earlier of other parameters which have been identified as coronary risk factors. For example, one relatively little publicized variable is serum uric acid level (figure 2-5).[7] There is a twofold increment in subjects with 7.0+ mg. percent versus <4.0 mg. percent. The prognostic utility of serum uric acid will be considered elsewhere (chapters 7, 10). For the moment it is safe to state that *uric acid is another predictor of coronary artery disease.*

Another significant single risk variable is emotional stress.[8] Figure 2-6 shows a twofold to a sixfold increase in the

13

percentage of coronary prevalence for high stress professional positions. The authors classify dermatologists, orthodontists, patent lawyers, and periodontists as "low" stress professional occupations. They denote "medium" stress for oral surgeons, other lawyers, pathologists, security analysts, and trial lawyers. The "high" stress professionals are stated to be anesthesiologists, general practice dentists, general practice physicians, and security traders.

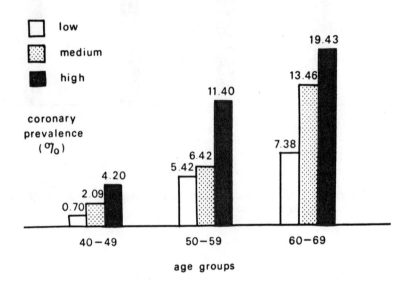

Russek, H.I. and Russek L.G. Etiologic factors in ischemic heart disease: the elusive role of emotional stress. Geriatrics 27: #1, 81–86, January 1972.

Figure 2-6. The relationship of age (expressed on the x-axis) and percentage of coronary prevalence (pictured on the y-axis) in terms of occupations according to stress.

Combination of Variables. Earlier reference was made to the fact that the incidence of coronary artery disease is increased more than fourfold in subjects with high versus low cholesterol levels irrespective of other risk factors (figure 2-2). Mention was made that the occurrence of coronary artery disease is fourfold in heavy smokers versus ex-smokers irrespective of other variables (figure 2-4). An examination of the *combination* of tobacco consumption *and* serum cholesterol is illustrated (figure 2-7).[9] In the nonsmoker with a serum cholesterol below 225 mg. percent, the incidence is one-half of one percent. In the smoker with a serum cholesterol of 275 mg. percent, the incidence is 8 percent.

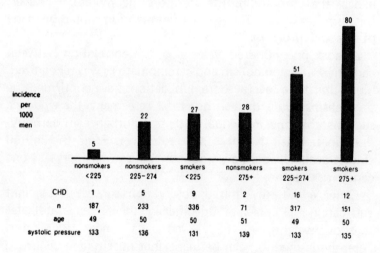

	nonsmokers <225	nonsmokers 225–274	smokers <225	nonsmokers 275+	smokers 225–274	smokers 275+
CHD	1	5	9	2	16	12
n	187	233	336	71	317	151
age	49	50	50	51	49	50
systolic pressure	133	136	131	139	133	135

People's Gas, Light, and Coke Company study, 1958-1962.

Figure 2-7. The incidence of clinical coronary heart disease in terms of tobacco consumption *and* serum cholesterol level.

Hence, the risk increase is sixteenfold. *The point being made is that, as one creates a coronary proneness profile with progressively more variables, the risk and thus the prediction increases and sharpens significantly.*

Cancer Proneness Profile

There is no question but that, in the field of proneness profiles, more energy and money have been expended to study coronary artery disease than any other single syndrome. It is, therefore, not at all surprising to find that the coronary proneness profile is more complete and has greater utility than any other profile.

Limited work is being carried on in other areas. It follows, hence, that the end-results are more incomplete. However, for purposes of this discussion, brief mention should be made of one such program.

Almost one hundred years ago[10] a correlation between carbohydrate metabolism and carcinomatosis was recognized. Since that time several score publications have confirmed the parallelism. While there is not total agreement, the evidence suggests that the individual with a disturbance in carbohydrate metabolism is more prone to cancer. From the limited studies available, carbohydrate metabolism may serve as one cancer risk factor.

Other, admittedly limited, observations suggest that weight and carcinoma correlate. Specifically, the evidence indicates that overweight may be viewed as a cancer risk factor. Parenthetic mention can be made that obesity and disturbed carbohydrate metabolism are also intimately related. Three observations are reported here simply to demonstrate the evidence which is already available.

Figure 2-8 portrays the two-hour postprandial blood sugar and blood glucose scores of 40 policemen and firemen who, as far as can be determined, are cancer-free. However, 20 report a family history of cancer; the remaining 20 have a negative familial story. On a mean difference basis, the blood

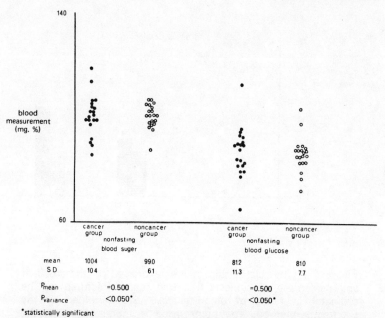

Figure 2-8. Comparison of nonfasting blood sugar and glucose levels in noncancer subjects with and without a familial history of cancer. The means are not significantly different in any of the groups. However, the variance is significant suggesting greater variability in blood sugar and glucose in noncancer subjects with a positive familial history of cancer.

sugar and blood glucose values are not statistically significant. However, the variance is significant (P <0.05). This suggests that there is greater blood glucose variability in noncancer subjects with a *positive* familial cancer history than in noncancer subjects with a *negative* familial history. *Phrased another way, individuals with a positive family cancer history have more variability in blood sugar, thus more relative hypo- and hyperglycemia.*[10]

A second study (figure 2-9) adds credence to the thesis that variations in carbohydrate metabolism and carcinomatosis correlate. It can be seen that the subjects reporting cancer show, with advancing age, higher blood glucose scores.[11]

17

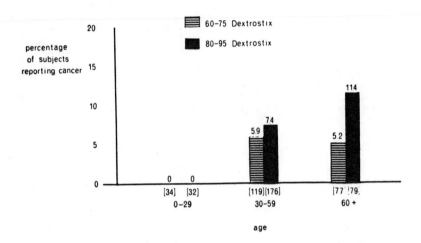

Figure 2-9. The relationship of age (expressed on the abscissa) and percentage of subjects reporting cancer (pictured on the ordinate) in terms of blood glucose as determined by the Dextrostix method. The point made is that, with time, the frequency of reported cancer is progressively higher in the subjects with the slightly higher blood glucose (black columns) irrespective of other variables.

Independent of blood glucose, in this same group, the heavier individuals report more cancer (figure 2-10). Finally, the incidence of cancer is brought into sharper focus when viewed in terms of *both* weight *and* blood glucose (figure 2-11). *Thus, the limited evidence implies that both increased weight and elevated blood glucose levels may be viewed as cancer risk factors and used in the development of a cancer proneness profile.*

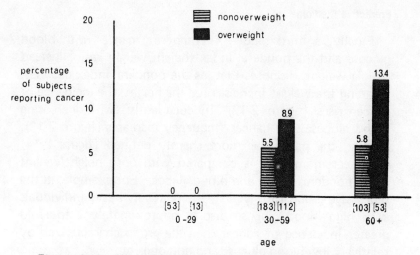

Figure 2-10. The relationship of age (on the x-axis) versus percentage of subjects reporting cancer (on the y-axis) in terms of weight. The point emphasized is that, with advancing age, the frequency of reported cancer is progressively higher in the overweight group (black columns) irrespective of other factors.

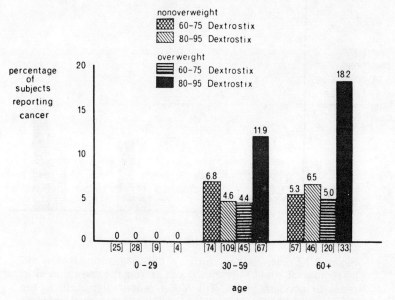

Figure 2-11. The relationship of age (on the horizontal axis) and percentage of subjects reporting cancer (on the vertical axis) in terms of weight and blood glucose. The overweight subjects with the slightly elevated blood glucose (black columns) show the highest rate.

Finally, a third report,[1 2] comparing cancer with blood glucose and the ponderal index (height/weight ratio) instead of just weight, discloses that, as the ponderal index declines, meaning the weight increases for the height, the incidence of cancer rises (figure 2-12). Independently, with increasing blood glucose, the cancer frequency increases (figure 2-13). Finally, the pattern is more sharply defined (figure 2-14) when carcinomatosis is compared with *both* height/weight ratio (ponderal index) *and* blood glucose. For example, in the oldest age group (50+ years), the relatively heavy individuals with high blood glucose display approximately a fourfold greater incidence of cancer than the group characterized by relatively low blood glucose and non-obesity.

Additional details regarding biochemical parameters in the cancer proneness profile will be provided in chapter 5.

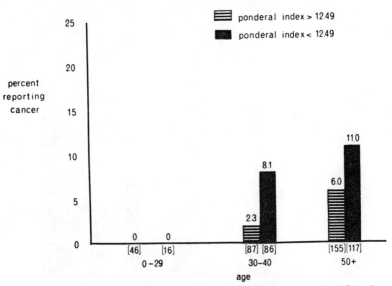

Figure 2-12. The relationship of age (on the horizontal axis) and percentage of subjects reporting cancer (on the vertical axis) in terms of ponderal index. The higher cancer rates occur in the subjects with the lower ponderal index (black columns), meaning the heavier individuals irrespective of other factors.

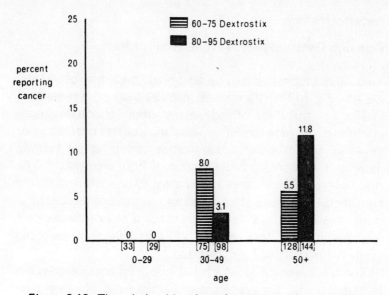

Figure 2-13. The relationship of age (on the x-axis) and percent of cancer subjects (on the y-axis) in terms of blood glucose. In the oldest age group, the highest incidence occurs in those with the higher blood glucose (black columns) irrespective of other variables.

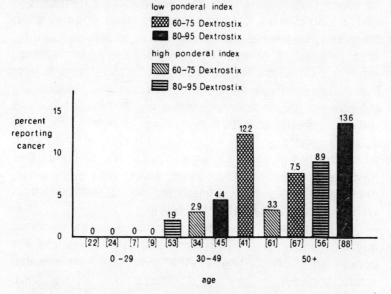

Figure 2-14. A comparison of age (on the abscissa) versus percent of subjects reporting cancer (on the ordinate) in terms of ponderal index and blood glucose. In the oldest age category, the highest rate is noted in subjects with the elevated blood glucose and low ponderal index (black columns).

Common Denominators in Proneness Profiles

Two illustrations, one well-advanced and the other less well-developed,[13] of proneness profiles have been presented. Obviously, there are already many other reasonably well-established parameters in these and other profiles. For example, the prognostic significance of the apical systolic murmur has been studied in terms of insurance risk.[14] The risk factors in the mother with regard to premature birth are published.[15] College attendance and serum urate concentrations have been correlated.[16] Proteinuria as a predictive tool is under study.[17] Maternal age and mongolism and leukemia in the offspring have been analyzed.[18]

The remaining point which has not been considered is the fact that many parameters are characteristic of more than one proneness profile. For example, impaired glucose tolerance has been demonstrated in a variety of apparently nondiabetic clinical disorders. Among these are psychopathies, cancer, hypertension, hyperlipidemias, atherosclerosis and arteriosclerosis, coronary heart disease, obesity, gout, pregnancy, congenital malformations or anomalies, sterility, drug suppression of ovulation, eye disorders, dermatitides, infectious states, multiple sclerosis, peptic ulcer, renal failure, liver disease, hyperthyroidism, osteoporosis, pulmonary emphysema, tic douloureux, and aging.[19] Also, at least 16 distinct genetic disorders (including Werner's syndrome, Turner's syndrome, and Alstrom's syndrome) are associated with impaired glucose tolerance.[20] Actually, this and other evidence implicates syndromes associated with every tissue, organ, and system which has been studied with regard to variations in carbohydrate metabolism.

One investigator has stated that impaired glucose tolerance might be expected to be present in 30 to 40 percent of the population.[21] According to this researcher, an elevated serum triglyceride level is a feature of diabetes, gout, atherosclerosis, and obesity. He concludes that "the association between impaired carbohydrate metabolism and athero-sclerosis, and between dietary carbohydrate [sucrose] and hypertriglyceridemia, and the increased triglyceride concen-tration accompanying hyperuricemia, are consistent with the hypothesis that the genetically associated diseases of gout, diabetes, atherosclerosis, and obesity are causally related to carbohydrate [sucrose] induced or aggravated hypertri-glyceridemia."

Summary

The susceptibility to certain diseases can be identified by the proneness profile technique. The prognostic parameters include such factors as age, family history, sex, weight, blood pressure, blood biochemical values, and dietary habits. Additional variables coming into focus are physical fitness, pollution, family situation, and occupation.

It is a well-known clinical fact, for example, that individ-uals with one chronic disorder sooner or later develop other chronic ailments.[22] This is clearly shown by similar clinical and biochemical findings. It would logically follow that there may be common denominators in seemingly different prone-ness profiles. This is shown through a discussion of the well-developed coronary proneness profile and the developing cancer proneness profile. In the final analysis, for predictive purposes, what is urgently needed is a proneness profile designed to anticipate the *syndrome of sickness,* a subject clarified in chapter 4.

References

1. Cheraskin, E. and Ringsdorf, W. M., Jr. *Predictive medicine: II. Experimental models.* J. Amer. Geriat. Soc. 19:5, 448-459, May 1971.

2. Stamler, J., Berkson, D. M., Levinson, M., Lindberg, H. A., Mojonnier, L., Miller, W. A., Hall, Y., and Andelman, S. L. *Coronary artery disease: status of preventive efforts.* Arch. Environ. Health 13:3, 322-335, September 1966.

3. Keys, A. *The individual risk of coronary heart disease.* Ann. New York Acad. Sc. 134:2, 1046-1056, 28 February 1966.

4. Stamler, J., Berkson, D. M., Lindberg, H. A., Hall, Y., Miller, W. A., Mojonnier, L., Levinson, M., Cohen, D. B., and Young, Q. D. *Coronary risk factors: their impact, and their therapy in the prevention of coronary heart disease.* Med. Clin. N. America 50:1, 229-254, January 1966.

Predictive Medicine

5. Stamler, J. *Atherosclerotic coronary heart disease: the major challenge to contemporary public health and preventive medicine.* Conn. Med. 28:9, 675-692, September 1964.

6. Stamler, J., Hall, Y., Mojonnier, L., Berkson, D. M., Levinson, M., Lindberg, H. A., Andelman, S. L., Miller, W. A., and Burkey, F. *Coronary proneness and approaches to preventing heart attacks.* Amer. J. Nursing 66:8, 1788-1793, August 1966.

7. Gertler, M. M., White, P. D., Cady, L. D., and Whiter, H. H. *Coronary heart disease: a prospective study.* Amer. J. Med. Sc. 248:4, 377-398, October 1964.

8. Russek, H. I. and Russek, L. G. *Etiological factors in ischemic heart disease: the elusive role of emotional stress.* Geriatrics 27:1, 81-86, January 1972.

9. Stamler, J. *Lectures on preventive cardiology.* 1967. New York, Grune and Stratton.

10. Cheraskin, E. and Ringsdorf, W. M., Jr. *Carbohydrate metabolism and carcinomatosis.* Cancer 17:2, 159-162, February 1964.

11. Cheraskin, E., Ringsdorf, W. M., Jr., Setyaadmadja, A. T. S. H., Barrett, R. A., Aspray, D. W., and Curry, S. *Cancer proneness profile: a study in weight and blood glucose.* Geriatrics 23:4, 134-137, April 1968.

12. Cheraskin, E., Ringsdorf, W. M., Jr., and Aspray, D. W. *Cancer proneness profile: a study in ponderal index and blood glucose.* Geriatrics 24:8, 121-125, August 1969.

13. Casey, A. E., Downey, E. L., Casey, J. G., Gilbert, F. E., and Thomason, S. *Detection of the cancer prone by the automated-computerized metabolic profile.* Ala. J. Med. Sc. 7:4, 375-384, October 1970.

14. Brown, H. B. *The prognostic significance of the apical systolic murmur from the insurance point of view.* Prog. Cardiovasc. Dis. 5:4, 329-334, January 1963.

15. Griswold, D. M. and Cavanagh, D. *Prematurity: the epidemiologic profile of the "high risk" mother.* Amer. J. Obst. Gynec. 96:6, 878-882, 15 November 1966.

16. Kasl, S. V., Brooks, G. W., and Cobb, S. *Serum urate concentrations in male high school students: a predictor of college attendance.* J. A. M. A. 198:7, 713-716, 14 November 1966.

17. Levitt, J. I. *The prognostic significance of proteinuria in young college students.* Ann. Int. Med. 66:4, 685-696, April 1967.

18. Stark, C. R. and Mantel, N. *Effects of maternal age and birth order on the risk of mongolism and leukemia.* J. Nat. Cancer Inst. 37:5, 687-698, November 1966.

19. Cheraskin, E. and Ringsdorf, W. M., Jr., *Diabetic dilemma in dentistry.* Acta Diabetologica Latina 8:2, 228-277, March-April 1971.

20. Editorial. *Diabetes mellitus: disease or syndrome?* The Lancet 1:7699, 583-584, 20 March 1971.

21. Ishmael, W. K. *Atherosclerotic vascular disease in familial gout, diabetes and obestiy.* Med. Times 94:2, 157-162, February 1966.

22. Cheraskin, E., Ringsdorf, W. M., Jr., and Clark, J. W. *Diet and disease.* 1968. Emmaus, Pennsylvania, Rodale Books. pp. 306-323.

An Ecologic Approach

It is as though I had on a table three dolls, one of glass, another of celluloid, and a third of steel, and I chose to hit the three dolls with a hammer, using equal strength. The first doll would break, the second would scar and the third would emit a pleasant musical sound.　　　　　　　　　　　　　—Jacques May.

Chapter 1 was relegated to a definition of a philosophy of health and disease called *predictive medicine*. The major point made was that there is a need for a system designed to *anticipate* rather than to *identify* disease. Chapter 2 demonstrated that *proneness profiles* are already feasible. Some are highly developed; others require additional investigation.

The purpose of this and subsequent chapters is to sketch the unusual or unique characteristics of predictive medicine. The immediate concern is to point up the utility of an ecologic approach to a predictive medicine program.[1]

Multifactorial Basis of Health and Disease

Earlier mention was made (chapter 1) that the history of medicine may be viewed in three phases. Originally disease was ascribed to a disturbance of the internal milieu. With the advent of the germ theory, the principal attention was shifted to the external world. In recent times the pendulum is swinging back to a midpoint between these concepts. It is now appreciated that, to produce disease, there must be an environmental challenge. However, whether man succumbs to the external threat is a function of his body's capacity to tolerate the external bombardment. This suggests that the formula for health and disease must be multifactorial.[2-7] Clearly, then, one does not by chance "catch a cold." In reality, it is the susceptible *soil* (body) of the organism that invites the ingress of the *seed* (virus). The obvious conclusion is that a realistic predictive medicine program must cope with *both* the environment and the host state.

Host Resistance and Susceptibility

The capacity of man to tolerate the environment has been variously termed *constitution, tissue tolerance, predisposition, secondary, systemic, intrinsic, and contributory factors.* Perhaps *host resistance and susceptibility* are the most popular terms for characterizing the state. Much remains to be elucidated about the ingredients which enter into host resistance and susceptibility. Notwithstanding, the ability of the organism to survive many and diverse external threats can be enhanced or worsened in a number of different ways. Among the many who have addressed themselves to this problem, Schneider describes the problem most lucidly:

"Resistance and susceptibility, in the minds of many, are relative terms applying to the same overall phenomenon, infection, and merely point to different ends of the same scale of events as they occur in the infected host. In this view, for example, 'more resistant' and 'less susceptible' are equivalent, interchangeable, and of equal usefulness. Indeed, as long as we are content to use these terms in making descriptive statements in comparing, say, one host with another, we are in no particular difficulties. For simplicity let us say Host A has survived and Host B has died. It matters little whether we say 'Host A is less susceptible than Host B,' or 'Host A is more resistant than Host B.' "[8]

But Schneider is not content to regard resistance and susceptibility in just a *descriptive* frame. His *analytic* approach contributes new light on these terms. He makes two cardinal points. First, host resistance and susceptibility are not simply antonyms. Second, host state may be modified in four ways: (1) by supplying an agent which enhances the host potential, (2) by adding an agent which diminishes host capacity, (3) by depriving the organism of an agent which enhances host capacity, and (4) by deprivation of an agent which diminishes host potential. The four possibilities can be readily demonstrated by many examples. When one supplies a child with sucrose, one invites the possibility of dental caries. This is item number two above. Conversely, the elimination of sucrose reduces the risk of dental decay. Here is an illustration of item number three. Hence, by definition, sucrose may be regarded as a *susceptibility* factor. Conversely, when one deprives the organism of vitamin C, one encourages capillary fragility, permeability, and bleeding (item number four). The addition of vitamin C minimizes the risk of capillary disruption and possible bleeding. This is illustrated by item number one. Thus, vitamin C becomes, by definition, a *resistance* factor. A workable predictive medicine program must recognize this concept, must ferret out the susceptibility and resistance variables, and must develop corrective measures.

The Resistance Factor. A number of agents may be identified as resistance variables in that their addition *reduces* the risk of illness and their subtraction *invites* disease. Thus, vitamins, minerals, proteins, essential fatty acids, enzymes, and other vital substances qualify as such agents. This subject will be developed in chapters 9 and 14.

Physical activity also qualifies as a resistance factor. To underline this point, 208 dentists and their wives completed the Cornell Medical Index Health Questionnaire.[9] The total number of affirmative responses in the M-R section is recognized as one barometer of psychologic state. The number of affirmative responses is the psychologic score which is in parallel with the psychologic state. Additionally, each subject indicated whether he or she engages in some form of exercise on a daily basis. Figure 3-1 pictorially portrays the results. It will be observed that the mean psychologic score is 3.0 for the 126 persons who report daily exercise. In contrast, the average score is 4.3 in the 82

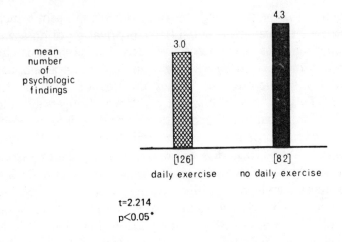

t=2.214
p<0.05*

*statistically significant difference of the means

Figure 3-1. The relationship of psychologic scores in terms of daily exercise. Those subjects with no daily exercise (black column) show a statistically significantly higher mean psychologic value irrespective of other variables.

persons who take no daily exercise. Thus, on a mean basis, the nonexercise group has a higher mean score by about 33 percent. Also, the difference is statistically significant [r = 2.214, P <0.05]. Thus, within the limits of these observations, it appears that there is a relationship between exercise and psychologic state.[1] What is relevant to this discussion is that, by definition, exercise may be viewed as a *resistance* factor.

Finally, from this and other evidence, it appears that a resistance factor for one disease or syndrome (e.g., exercise and coronary artery disease) is very likely a resistance factor for other disorders (e.g., exercise and abnormal psychologic state). More attention will be directed to this point at a later time (chapters 9, 10, 14).

It should be pointed out that the relationship between a resistance agent and health is parabolic. For example, too little exercise allows the health status to worsen, and excessive physical activity may produce illness. The proper amount, however, will promote good health.

The Susceptibility Factor. A number of factors may be identified as susceptibility agents in that their addition *increases* the risk of disease and their subtraction *minimizes* the possibility of illness. As previously cited, dietary sucrose qualifies as a susceptibility agent. Other dietary factors are highly saturated fats, extensively refined (processed) carbohydrate from the cereal grains, chemical additives and contaminents in foods, and alcohol. There is increasing interest in the role of pollutants in the air and water as susceptibility agents.

Frequently overlooked dietary factors are coffee and tea.[10] To analyze this point, the 208 dentists and their wives previously mentioned were also classified in terms of daily coffee/tea intake (figure 3-2).[1] The mean psychologic score is 3.0 for those consuming less than three cups of coffee and/or tea daily. In contrast, the average psychologic score is 50 percent worse [4.5] for the group characterized by the higher coffee/tea intake. Finally, the difference is statistically significant ($t = 2.238$, $P < 0.025$). The major point is that, within the limits of this study and others, excessive coffee/tea consumption may be viewed as a *susceptibility* factor. What is also significant is that coffee/tea intake is relatively unrecognized in its possible role in host resistance and susceptibility.[11-13] More specific consideration will be accorded to the susceptibility aspects of health and disease in chapters 9, 10, 14.

The Resistance-susceptibility Constellation

The isolated examples of host resistance and susceptibility just cited, while interesting, do not present the complete picture. Actually, to repeat, health and disease are multifactorial in nature. Thus, they are the net result of *many* resistance and susceptibility agents. To underline this point,

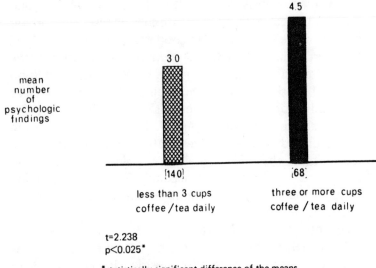

Figure 3-2. The relationship of psychologic scores in terms of daily coffee/tea consumption. Those subjects consuming the greater quantities of coffee/tea (black column) show a statistically significantly higher mean psychologic value, irrespective of other variables.

figure 3-3 relates psychologic state to one resistance (exercise) and one susceptibility (coffee/tea) factor singly and in combination. It is noteworthy that the lowest mean psychologic score (2.6) is observed in the group taking daily exercise (high resistance) and not consuming appreciable amounts of coffee/tea (low susceptibility). It is equally significant that the highest average psychologic score (4.9), almost double the lowest, occurs in the group with no daily exercise (low resistance) *and* consuming greater amounts of coffee/tea (high susceptibility). Figure 3-3 also shows that these two groups differ significantly (t = 2.522, P <0.025). Finally, the two intermediate groups, in terms of resistance and susceptibility, occupy intermediate positions with regard to psychologic state.

Resistance and susceptibility factors are so interrelated that one may serve to cancel out or reduce the effects of another. For example, laboratory tests on rats have shown that those fortified with vitamin E (resistance agent) live

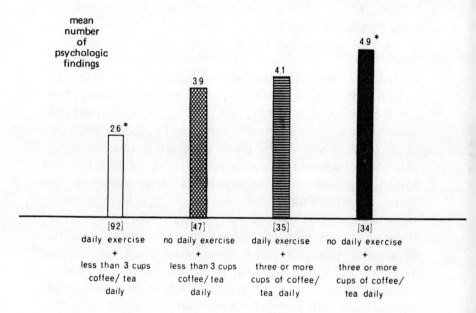

*statistically significant difference of the means [t=2.522, p<0.025]

Figure 3-3. The relationship of psychologic scores in terms of daily exercise and coffee/tea consumption. The group with no daily exercise and consuming the greater amounts of coffee/tea (black column) show a statistically significantly higher mean score than the group with daily exercise and relatively less coffee/tea consumption (white column).

twice as long as those not treated with vitamin E in an atmosphere which simulates smog concentrations comparable to those found over Los Angeles or Tokyo (susceptibility agent).[14]

From these limited results it appears that vitamin E (resistance agent) is beneficial in protecting the lung from obstructive lung diseases such as emphysema and edema that are caused by smog (susceptibility agent). A further increase in air pollution, however, was observed to cancel out the improved resistance provided by vitamin E fortification. Vitamin E may also serve as a resistance agent in cardiovascular disease (chapter 14).

Summary

In the final analysis, whether one succumbs to disease or remains unscathed is a function of the world one lives in and one's capacity to withstand the external bombardment. As Jacques May[15] has so eloquently phrased it, some people are made of glass and shatter under the slightest environmental challenge. These are the people with a high degree of host susceptibility and poor resistance. Others appear to be structured of celluloid and only scar. Some few are structured of steel and tolerate well the outer world. These are those with good host resistance and a low host susceptibility. A practical predictive medicine program must take cognizance of the internal milieu, and must identify and alter those variables which contribute to the body's resistance and susceptibility. Only in this manner can one confer upon the glass doll the characteristics of steel and, hopefully, at least produce a better fabric of man.

References

1. Cheraskin, E. and Ringsdorf, W. M., Jr. *Predictive medicine: III. An ecologic approach.* J. Amer. Geriat. Soc. 19:6, 505-510, June 1971.

2. Cheraskin, E., Ringsdorf, W. M., Jr., and Clark, J. W. *Diet and disease.* 1968. Emmaus, Pennsylvania, Rodale Books, Inc.

3. Wylie, C. M. *The definition and measurement of health and disease.* Pub. Health Rep. 85:2, 100-104, February 1970.

4. Elsom, K. O. *Elements of the medical process; their place in medical care planning.* J. A. M. A. 217:9, 1226-1232, 30 August, 1971.

5. Hoyman, H. S. *An ecologic view of health and health education.* J. School Health 35:3, 110-123, March 1965.

6. Fitzgerald, R. J. and Keyes, P. H. *Dental caries as a major disease problem.* Med. Ann. D. C. 34:10, 463-467, October 1965.

7. Scrimshaw, N. S. *Ecological factors in nutritional disease.* Amer. J. Clin. Nutrit. 14:2, 112-122, February 1964.

8. Schneider, H. S. *Nutrition and resistance-susceptibility to infection.* Amer. J. Trop. Med. 31:2, 174-182, March 1951.

9. Brodman, K., Erdman, A. J., Jr., and Wolff, H. G. *Cornell Medical Index Health Questionnaire.* 1949. New York, Cornell University Medical College.

10. Cheraskin, E., Ringsdorf, W. M., Jr., Setyaadmadja, A. T. S. H., and Barrett, R. A. *Blood glucose levels after caffeine.* Lancet 2:7569, 689, 21 September 1968.

11. Jankelson, O. M., Beaser, S. B., Howard, F. M., and Mayer, J. *Effect of coffee on glucose tolerance and circulating insulin in men with maturity-onset diabetes.* Lancet 1:7489, 527-529, 11 March 1967.

12. Albertson, P. *How much coffee can your heart take?* Pageant, pp. 39-44, March 1968.

13. Medical News. *Coffee's effect on diabetes tested.* J. A. M. A. 209:3, 350, 21 July 1969.

14. *Dietary drugs limit pollution ills.* U. S. Medicine 6:4, 1 September 1970.

15. May, J. M. *The ecology of human disease.* Ann. New York Acad. Sc. 84:17, 789-794, 8 December 1960.

The Gradation Concept

The researchers took as their hypothesis the concept that health and disease are not absolutes, but occur in a spectrum ranging from perfect health to death. . . . "We have been thinking that the time has come to speak in terms of percentage of disease," Danowski said. "For example, some people have difficulty holding down their weight. Some of these people may have 14 percent Cushing's disease. Yet, by present techniques, they might not be detected." —T. S. Danowski.

In chapter 3 the point was made that one of the unique features of a predictive medicine program is that it recognizes the multifactorial pattern of health and disease and seeks to identify the factors which contribute to host resistance and susceptibility. This chapter is designed to demonstrate another special feature of predictive medicine. Specifically, it will show its awareness of the fact that health and disease occur in gradations,[1] which may be pictured in an achromatic series, utilizing white and black as limiting poles.[2] This suggests a spectrum of an infinite number of shades of gray interposed between the limiting end points. It is in this gray area that predictive medicine finds its greatest utility in the *anticipation* rather than simply the *identification* of disease.

Organizations devoted to prevention of disease must adopt the principles of predictive medicine if their goals are to be reached. Recently, the Board of Regents of the American College of Preventive Medicine issued this official definition of their organization: "Preventive medicine is that branch of medicine which has primary interest in preventing physical, mental, and emotional disease and injury in contrast to treating the sick and injured. Secondarily, it is concerned with slowing the progress of disease and conserving maximal function."[3]

34

Only through prediction or anticipation of disease, however, can such purposes be fulfilled and primary prevention (prevention of occurrence) be effectively achieved.

The Course of Disease

All disease is preceded by an incubation period. In the instance of acute mechanical trauma (e.g., an automobile accident) the incubation time is too brief for predictive purposes. In the case of acute infectious disorders (e.g., measles) the incubation period is somewhat longer (e.g., approximately ten days) and more significant from a prognosticative standpoint. With the chronic disorders (e.g., myocardial infarction, cerebrovascular accident, rheumatoid arthritis, periodontal disease) the incubation time extends over months and frequently several years or decades. For example, the vasculature may reveal degenerative changes as early as the first year of life. Clearly, the longer the period, the greater the opportunity to anticipate the problem and end it and, hopefully, abort the process. In order to effect primary prevention (prevention of occurrence) as described in chapter 1, it is necessary to analyze the sequence of events which eventuates in classical disease syndromes.

Initially the patient notes only few and seemingly unrelated findings.[4] There may be irritability, for example, associated with leg cramps. Because these apparently unrelated symptoms and signs do not fit any textbook description of a particular disease, the complaints may either be ignored, assigned a meaningless label, or regarded as a minor psychic problem and treated symptomatically. The latter diagnosis is frequently made by exclusion. In other words, a failure to relate the signs and symptoms to classical disease nomenclature usually results in the decision that the problem is likely an emotional one. At this stage, the clinical picture is shown by the box on the left (figure 4-1). This area will be enlarged upon in chapter 11.

If the clinical situation just described continues, as is so often the case, then the number of symptoms and signs progressively multiplies. Sooner or later the findings begin to crystallize in systems, organs, or in localized sites. For

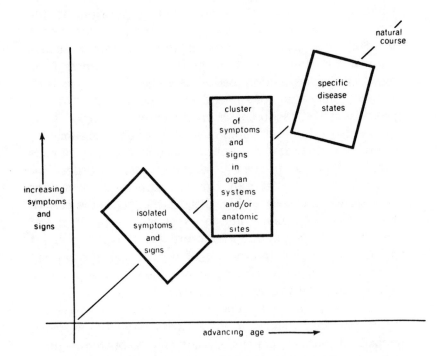

Figure 4-1. The clinical sequence of events in chronic disease. At first, there are few and diverse symptoms and findings (box on the left). With time, the findings become more numerous and localized in a system or organ (middle box). Finally, the clinical evidence fits the textbook picture of a particular disease or syndrome (box on the right).

instance, a subject may find himself with several gastrointestinal complaints (e.g., indigestion, anorexia, and hemorrhoids). At this stage, the constellation is still not classifiable with textbook disease terminology. Hence, treatment is usually symptomatic and/or the patient is advised that the problem should be under observation. If many organ systems and/or anatomic sites are involved, the syndrome might be ascribed a psychologic etiology. This is the story shown in the middle box (figure 4-1). This phase in the genesis of disease will be discussed in greater detail in chapter 11. Finally, when the syndrome is clearly identifiable in terms of its classical description, then the illness is assigned a label. In conventional medicine, it is only at this point that a diagnosis is deemed justifiable. This is pictorially portrayed in the box on the right (figure 4-1). Even at this stage, however, the interrelationships between several existing diseases are frequently overlooked (see chapter 11).

The gradation concept has long been recognized. The following citation is representative of the thinking: One has little difficulty in distinguishing between life and death, but the distinction between illness and health is not an easy one to make. Except for certain acute illnesses the transition from health to ill health is often imperceptible. A useful approach is to view health as a spectrum. This spectrum ranges from perfect health to the complete absence of health, or death. Between these two extremes there is little agreement on criteria for differentiating the various degrees of ill health. Nevertheless, the need to make these distinctions has been growing in recent years.[5]

According to Robert M. Thorner of the National Center for Health Services Research and Development [HEW, Rockville, Maryland], there are seven stages in the natural history of untreated disease in an individual: (1) birth, (2) exposure to risk, (3) precursory physiologic changes, (4) early symptoms, (5) frank but not disabling illness, (6) disabling illness, and (7) death.[6]

Prevention of recurrence (secondary prevention) may be accomplished by applying preventive techniques during stages five and six. However, primary prevention or prevention of occurrence must take place much earlier. Effective primary prevention can only be achieved through the application of *predictive medicine.*

The Clinical Course of Events

The story just described can be simply demonstrated.[2] One thousand two hundred twenty-four presumably healthy female subjects completed the Cornell Medical Index Health Questionnaire.[7] Section D, consisting of 23 questions, relates to the gastrointestinal tract. Figure 4-2 compares age (on the horizontal axis) with the frequency of reported gastrointestinal symptoms and signs (on the vertical axis). Four points warrant special attention. First, with advancing age the *mean* number of gastrointestinal findings increases (2.9 to 3.2 to 3.5). Second, in the oldest age group (70-89 years) the average number of findings declines (3.5 to 3.1). Third, with advancing age the variance generally widens. Fourth, in the oldest age group the variance shrinks.

This simple experiment is a clinical expression of the pattern earlier presented (figure 4-1) showing the usual course of events in the genesis of disease states. In the early years the symptoms and signs are relatively few and usually so diverse that the total picture does not lend itself for a classical textbook diagnosis (e.g., peptic ulcer). With advancing time, the findings increase in number and begin to localize in systems and sites. Finally, the constellation fits the classical requirements for a particular disease tag.

The gradation concept is an important and integral part of a predictive medicine program. Awareness of the course of events means that effort can be directed at an *early* stage to the number and pattern of symptoms and signs rather than simply waiting for the identification of a specific disease syndrome.

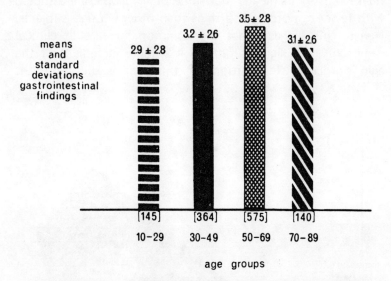

Figure 4-2. The relationship of age (on the x-axis) and frequency of reported gastrointestinal findings (on the y-axis). With age, up to a point, the mean number of symptoms and signs increases. After the age of seventy (the present life expectancy of man), the findings decline. With age, up to a point, the variance widens suggesting that some older subjects have fewer findings than young people. After the age of seventy, the variance declines.

The usual pictorial portrayal shows that, with advancing age, there is a progressive increase in symptoms and signs (figure 4-3). What is usually not underlined is that, with time, there is an increase in variance [shown by the gray area in figure 4-3]. This means that some older people are afflicted with fewer symptoms and signs than other younger subjects. Hence, this suggests that the common increase in clinical symptoms and signs is *not* an inevitable ingredient of the aging process. Recognition of this fact is an important

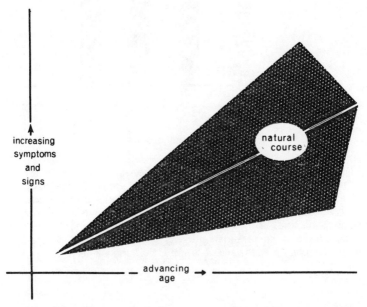

Figure 4-3. The usual clinical sequence of events. With time there is a progressive increase in symptoms and signs (shown by the rising center line). However, with advancing age there is also an increase in variance (pictured by the widening gray area). This suggests that some elderly persons show fewer findings than other younger individuals.

characteristic of a predictive medicine program, namely, that much of the clinical picture heretofore ascribed to the *physiologic* aging process is, in fact, simply an expression of pathosis. That the usual aging course of events is not physiologic allows that the process may be slowed, stopped, reversed, or even completely prevented (figure 4-4).[8] The latter, prevention of occurrence, however, must begin early in life. Thus, in reality, most chronic diseases are pediatric in origin.

Finally, it is noteworthy that in the eighth and ninth decades (the time beyond the current infant life expectancy of three score and ten) the mean number of findings and/or the variance may decline (figure 4-2). This is so because only the heartiest subjects (survival of the fittest) are still living. The ill have already succumbed. Parenthetic mention should be made that this characteristic of the aged will be discussed again as it relates to the oral cavity (chapter 12).

Awareness of this pattern plays a significant role in the philosophy of a predictive medicine program. These elderly living subjects, having already proved success, should be employed for the development of norms and standards of health (see chapter 6).

The Biochemical Course of Events

The pattern just outlined is not confined to the clinical state.[9] When other levels of health and disease are scrutinized, similar results follow. Figure 4-5 is a summary of fasting and nonfasting blood glucose scores, by the Dextrostix method, in 6,143 presumably healthy female subjects.[1] Shown are the age groups on the abscissa and the mean blood glucose scores and standard deviations on the ordinate. It is relevant that, with advancing age, the mean scores slowly but progressively rise. It is also interesting that, with time, the variances continue to increase. This suggests that some elderly persons have lower blood glucose levels than other younger people. However, as with clinical symp-

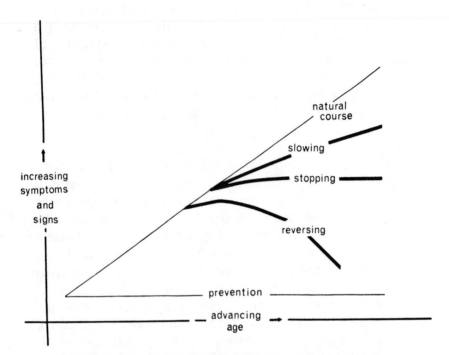

Figure 4-4. The five possible clinical events are shown. First, the clinical course continues unchanged. Second, the process may be slowed. Third, it is sometimes possible to stop the pattern. Fourth, there is a chance of reversing the state of affairs. Finally, the ideal is to subtend an angle of zero with real primary prevention (prevention of occurrence).

toms and signs, in the very elderly the variance begins to shrink.

Thus, norms established from the healthy young and aged can play a cardinal role in the philosophy of a predictive medicine program. This thesis reemphasizes the importance of the healthy aged group. It also underscores the fact that biochemical parameters from birth to death change very little in the healthy subject.

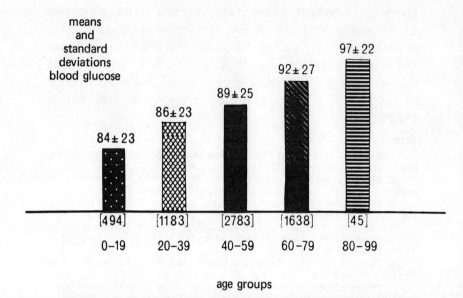

Figure 4-5. The relationship of age (on the abscissa) and blood glucose as measured by the Dextrostix method (on the ordinate). With advancing age the mean scores continue to rise. With advancing time the variances increase, indicating that some elderly people have lower blood glucose scores than other younger subjects. Finally, in older subjects the variance declines.

Summary

In the traditional practice of medicine, a diagnosis is only made when a set number and constellation of symptoms and signs prevail. Hence, for practical purposes, the long and tortuous incubation period, clinically and biochemically, goes frequently unlabeled or tagged as an ill-defined psychologic syndrome. Sensitivity to the clinical and biochemical events is an integral part of a predictive medicine plan. As

Predictive Medicine

Danowski[10] so aptly pointed out, it is time to think in terms of 20 percent of disease X and 40 percent of disease Y. This approach not only invites the earlier *identification* of disease but, more importantly, its *anticipation* with the institution of earlier therapy for primary prevention. Additional evidence in support of the gradation concept will be presented in chapter 5.

References

1. Elsom, K. O. *Elements of the medical process; their place in medical care planning.* J. A. M. A. 217:9, 1226-1232, 30 August 1971.

2. Cheraskin, E. and Ringsdorf, W. M., Jr. *Predictive medicine: IV. The gradation concept.* J. Amer. Geriat. Soc. 19:6, 511-516, June 1971.

3. Disease Detection Information Bureau. *American College of Preventive Medicine defines preventive medicine.* DDIB Newsletter 4:4, 16, September 1971.

4. Hammond, E. C. *Some preliminary findings on physical complaints from a prospective study of 1,064,004 men and women.* Amer. J. Pub. Health 54:1, 11-23, January 1964.

5. Rogers, E. S. *Human ecology and health.* 1960. New York, The Macmillan Company. pp. 167-174.

6. Disease Detection Information Bureau. *HEW official advises more caution, skepticism toward prevention 'panacea'.* DDIB Newsletter 4:4, 5, 11, September 1971.

7. Brodman, K., Erdman, A. J., Jr., and Wolff, H. G. *Cornell Medical Index Health Questionnaire.* 1949. New York, Cornell University Medical College.

8. Still, J. W. *Adult preventive medicine: the fourth phase in the evolution of medicine.* J. Amer. Geriat. Soc. 16:4, 395-406, April 1968.

9. Casey, A. E., Downey, E., and Selikoff, K. I. *Age changes in the metabolic profile.* Alabama J. Med. Sc. 6:3, 308-310, July 1969.

10. Danowski, T. S. and Moses, C., Jr. *Cholesterol levels reduced by hormone 'replacement doses.'* J. A. M. A. 181:9, 27-28, 1 September 1962.

Linear Versus Curvilinear Functions

He [Claude Bernard] emphasized that at all levels of biological organization, in plants as well as in animals, survival and fitness are conditioned by the ability of the organism to resist the impact of the outside world and maintain constant within narrow limits the physicochemical characteristics of its internal environment.   —Rene Dubos.

Earlier chapters have dealt with the philosophy of a predictive medicine program, its experimental models, the unique appreciation of ecologic principles, and recognition that health and disease exist in a spectrum. This chapter deals with another singular feature of predictive medicine, namely, its awareness of viewing parameters of health and disease as linear or curvilinear relationships.[1]

By act, if not by word, traditional medicine is based upon a philosophy that the relationship between different parameters with regard to health and disease is a linear function. For example, the higher the blood glucose the more pathologic is this particular biochemical barometer. This is abundantly exemplified[2] by the usual description of the genesis of diabetes mellitus (figure 5-1). At one point (on the extreme left) there is no hyperglycemia, no glycosuria, and no clinical findings. Subsequently, there is the appearance of hyperglycemia with no glycosuria or clinical symptoms and signs. As time progresses, however, hyperglycemia, glycosuria, and clinical symptoms and signs appear. It is at this point that, by definition, the patient is given a diagnosis of diabetes mellitus. Three items deserve special consideration.

45

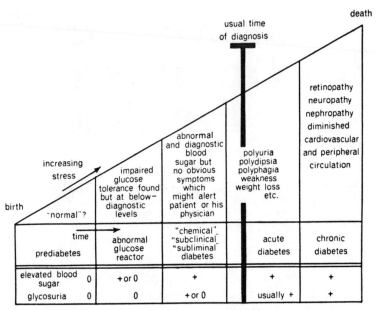

Krall,L.P. When is diabetes? Med. Clin. N. Amer. 49: #4,893–904,July 1965.

Figure 5-1. A classical clinical-biochemical description of the course of events in diabetes mellitus.

First, the sequence of events (figure 5-1) underscores the gradation concept described in chapter 4. Second, the story underlines the arbitrary delineation of health and sickness. Finally, the chart emphasizes one of the common characteristics of traditional medicine, namely, that many biochemical patterns are viewed as a dichotomy (hyper- versus normoglycemia). It is of parenthetic interest that, of all biochemical procedures in multiphasic screening programs, blood glucose is the second most commonly employed biochemical test.[3]

The simple fact of the matter is that, for predictive purposes, all biochemical parameters must be viewed as a trichotomy rather than a dichotomy. In the instance just cited (figure 5-1) recognition is given to hyperglycemia versus nonhyperglycemia, but no attention is accorded hypoglycemia even though the latter is recognized as a possible early diabetic sign.[4]

Mortality and the Curvilinear-linear Concept

A simple yet most graphic representation of the trichotomy concept has been published by Waters, Withey, Kilpatrick, Wood, and Abernethy.[5] They measured the packed cell volume (PCV) in 180 women in 1958 and reported the percentage of deaths in the group ten years later (figure 5-2).

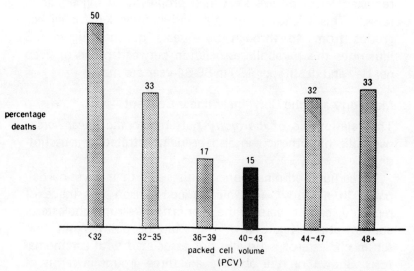

Waters, W.E., Withey, J.L., Kilpatrick, G.S. ,Wood, P.H.N. and Abernethy, M.
Ten-year haematological follow-up: mortality and haematological changes.
Brit. Med. Jour. 4: 761-764, 27 December 1969.

Figure 5-2. The curvilinear or parabolic relationship of mortality and packed cell volume depicting the optimal hematocrit as being in the middle.

Described on the abscissa are the hematocrit groups ranging (left to right) from the low to the high scores. Pictured on the ordinate are the percentage of deaths. It is abundantly evident that the highest mortality figures occur at *both* ends of the PCV scale. Also the chart shows that the individuals with the middle scores (in this case PCV of 40-43) are paralleled by the least mortality. It is well to point out that the hematocrit is the fourth most popularly utilized test in the approximately 120 operational multiple testing programs in the United States.[3]

Mortality and the curvilinear concept are not restricted to biochemical findings. For example, in a study of 1,064,004 men and women, those who reported about seven hours of sleep per night had the lowest death rates. Those who reported more or less sleep had progressively higher death rates.[6] This trichotomous relationship prevailed for all age groups from 45 through 85+ years of age. Figure 5-3 illustrates this parabolic association between hours of sleep per day and deaths per 100 in 80-84-year-old men.

Morbidity and the Curvilinear-linear Concept

The relationship of *morbidity* patterns to the linear versus parabolic hypothesis can also be demonstrated as a trichotomy.

Three hundred ninety-one dentists and their wives participated in a study[1] in which a comparison was made of reported cancer versus the nonfasting serum cholesterol concentration (figure 5-4). It should be pointed out that serum cholesterol is usually not associated with carcinomatosis. Shown on the abscissa are three groups in terms of nonfasting serum cholesterol. Described on the ordinate is the percentage of subjects reporting cancer. It will be noted that the pattern is essentially parabolic with the least reporting of cancer in the center group (200-250 mg. percent).

The degree of curvilinearity in this group is a function of a

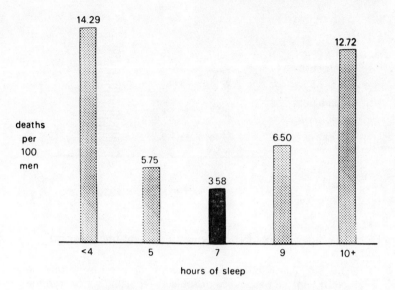

Hammond. E C Some preliminary findings on physical complaints from a prospective study of 1.064.004 men and women. Am. J. Public Health 54 #1,11-23. January 1964

Figure 5-3. The curvilinear or parabolic relationship of mortality and hours of sleep per day depicting the optimal sleep time of seven hours.

number of variables. Notably, the delineating points can be expressed in terms of serum cholesterol and the age factor.

Figure 5-5 describes the relationship between reported cancer and serum cholesterol in terms of age in the same sample. Two points are particularly noteworthy. First, the parabolic relationship between nonfasting serum cholesterol and the percentage of subjects reporting cancer does not exist in the relatively young group under 40 years of age (the stippled columns). Second, in the older group (40+ years of age) the curvilinear pattern is not only evident but with more

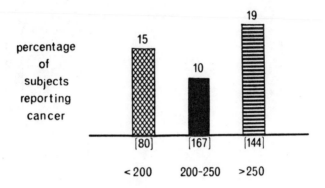

nonfasting serum cholesterol (mg. percent)

Figure 5-4. The relationship of serum cholesterol levels (on the abscissa) and the percentage of subjects reporting cancer (on the ordinate) irrespective of other variables. The lowest score (black column) is associated with the middle serum cholesterol group. Higher cancer figures occur in both the relative hypo- and hypercholesterolemia groups (stippled columns). This underscores the parabolic relationship of cancer and serum cholesterol.

graphic clarity than when the relationship of cholesterol and cancer is plotted irrespective of age (figure 5-4). Hence, the older the group, the more sharply defined is the parabolic pattern.

The degree of curvilinearity is also a function of the physiologic range of values established for a biochemical parameter. Figure 5-6 pictorially portrays the information shown in earlier illustrations. The one difference is that the middle group, in terms of serum cholesterol, is more restrictive (210-240 mg. percent) than in figure 5.5 (200-250 mg. percent). The evidence indicates, by this method, that the parabolic functions are more sharply defined. Thus, there is a suggestive curvilinear pattern in the young (under 40 years of age) in addition to a retention of the more sharply demarcated parabola in the older group (black columns).

Finally, to underscore the relationship between serum

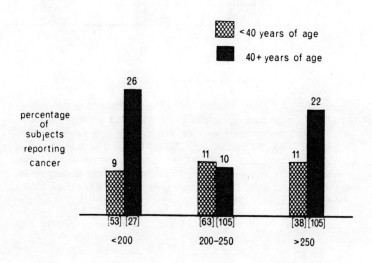

Figure 5-5. A comparison of serum cholesterol (on the x-axis) and percentage of subjects reporting cancer (on the y-axis) in terms of age. In the relatively young group (stippled columns) there appears to be no relationship. In sharp contrast, in the older age group (black columns) the parabolic configuration is clearly evident. Hence, the addition of the time factor influences the curvilinear picture.

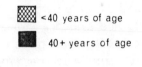

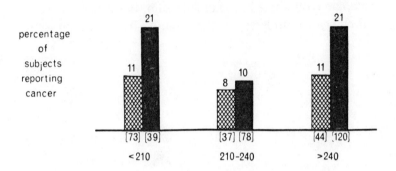

nonfasting serum cholesterol (mg. percent)

Figure 5-6. The correlation of serum cholesterol (on the horizontal axis) and percentage of reported cancer (on the vertical axis) in terms of a more restricted middle range (serum cholesterol 210-240 versus 200-250 in figure 5-4) and age. By constricting the area of relative normocholesterolemia, the younger group (stippled columns) begins to show a suggested parabola. However, in the relatively older category the curvilinear configuration is very clear.

cholesterol and cancer in terms of age *and* more restricted criteria for serum cholesterol, figure 5-7 is included. The one salient point is that, when the older age group is even older (<45 versus 45+ years) than earlier shown (<40 versus 40+ years in figure 5-5), the curvilinear arrangement is even more clearly outlined (black bars). The percentage reporting cancer is threefold greater in those with the lower and higher serum cholesterol values.

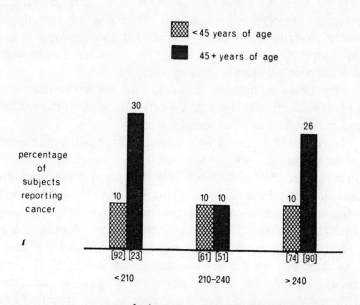

Figure 5-7. An analysis of the relationship of serum cholesterol with relative normocholesterolemia in a more restricted range (210-240 versus 200-250) shown on the abscissa and percentage of subjects reporting cancer depicted on the ordinate with an age delineation at a higher level (45+ versus 40+) than in earlier illustrations (figure 5-4 and 5-5). In this instance, the parabolic pattern in the older group (black columns) is more sharply defined than in any of the other categorizations.

Early Disease and the Curvilinear-linear Concept

These and the many other examples which could be cited demonstrate that health exists only in an atmosphere of homeostasis. The body, physiologically and metabolically, is designed to operate within a narrow range of fluctuation. Both increases or decreases in body functions or in its chemical constituents may signify the development of disease.

It is known, for example, that high and low blood pressure, hemoglobin, hematocrit, et cetera, are pathologic. Although little significance is accorded such variations as a low blood triglyceride, uric acid, or enzyme level, these must also be regarded as indicators of pathosis.

The parabolic pattern described with regard to mortality and classical morbidity (e.g., cancer) extends into the earliest and most subtle expressions of disease.

To illustrate this, 1,743 presumably healthy subjects[1] participating in the annual diabetes detection drive in Birmingham, Alabama, were selected. Each completed the Cornell Word Form-2 test.[7] This is a simple, self-administered, controlled association test designed to quantify psychic state. Figure 5-8 pictures the blood glucose scores (Dextrostix method) on the horizontal axis and the mean CWF-2 scores on the vertical scale. The lowest (3.3) score occurs in the middle (black bar) with rising values associated with *both* relative hyper- and hypoglycemia (stippled columns). This is particularly interesting in view of the fact that this parabolic pattern appears with no consideration given to the age factor and no special recognition accorded the time the blood sample was taken.

Summary

Traditional medicine, by act if not by word, views biochemical patterns in a *dichotomous* system. For example, serum cholesterol is judged to be either high or acceptable. Little or no significance is accorded hypocholesterolemia. A cardinal feature of a predictive medicine program is to view these systems as a *trichotomy* with hypo-, normo-, and hypercholesterolemia, hypo-, normo-, and hyperglycemia, et cetera.

In this chapter, the relationship of serum cholesterol and cancer was utilized as an experimental model to underline the parabolic concept. It should be pointed out that the curvilinear concept prevails in many other disease syndromes[8-22] and with many other biochemical

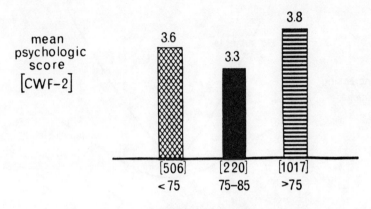

Figure 5-8. The parabolic relationship of blood glucose (on the abscissa) and mean psychologic scores (on the ordinate). The highest, the most pathologic scores are at both ends (stippled columns); the lowest and least pathologic findings are in the middle (black bar).

measures.[10-14,16,17,19-24] What is particularly noteworthy is that one arm of the parabola is frequently ignored.[25] Excellent examples are hypocholesterolemia and hypoglycemia.

The parabolic pattern is, in part, a function of age (figure 5-9). In the relatively young, the parabola is quite flat; with time the picture becomes more sharply defined. Thus, the biochemical-clinical parallelism must exist long enough to become demonstrable, and age is the essential time ingredient.

The curvilinear concept is not limited to biochemical

55

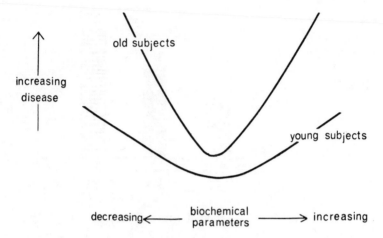

Figure 5-9. The relationship of health status and a biochemical parameter is curvilinear rather than linear as generally held. The parabolic pattern increases with advancing age.

parameters of health and disease. Clinical estimates or findings also conform to the parabolic pattern.[6] Figure 5-10 pictorializes the parabolic relationship between daily hours of sleep and mortality in men 50-54, 60-64, and 80-84 years of age. It is apparent that with time the curvilinear pattern is increasingly more defined.

Relationships between diet and disease readily demonstrate this parabolic phenomenon. Figure 5-11 points out that an increase in caries activity in 183 adults occurs when the dietary calcium/phosphorus ratio increases or decreases beyond a very narrow range.[26]

This parabolic phenomenon cancels out statistical significance with the t test. The mean dietary Ca/P ratio of 0.57 in

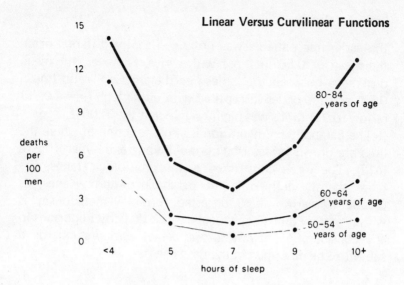

Hammond, E.C. Some preliminary findings on physical complaints from a prospective study of 1,064,004 men and women. Am. J. Public Health 54: #1, 11–23, January 1964

Figure 5-10. The relationship between health status and a clinical parameter. Death and hours of sleep present a curvilinear pattern. The parabola becomes more sharply defined as age increases.

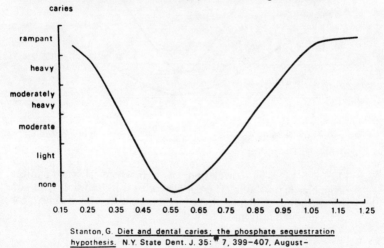

Stanton, G. Diet and dental caries; the phosphate sequestration hypothesis. N.Y. State Dent. J. 35: # 7, 399–407, August–September 1969.

Figure 5-11. Curvilinear relationship between dental caries and the dietary calcium/phosphorus ratio in 183 dental patients. Both an increase and a decrease in the dietary ratio is correlated with caries activity.

the caries-free patients was not significantly different from the mean of 0.56 in those with caries. However, the mean difference between the caries-free dietary Ca/P ratio (mean 0.57) and the caries-susceptible with either high (mean 0.79) or low (0.39) ratios was highly significant (P <0.001).

The parabolic configuration is also a function of where the lines are drawn to describe normo-, hypo-, and hyper- (figure 5-12). The more constricted is the physiologic range, the more sharply defined is the parabolic pattern. Hence, as Claude Bernard[27] has suggested, optimal metabolism is within narrow limits. This becomes particularly important in any consideration of *physiologic* versus *normal* standards, a subject to be described in the next chapter.

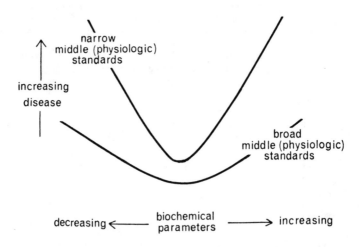

Figure 5-12. The correlation of a biochemical and clinical parameter is parabolic. The curvilinearity is in part a function of the definition of hyper-, hypo-, and normo- for the biochemical technique in question.

References

1. Cheraskin, E. and Ringsdorf, W. M., Jr. *Predictive medicine: V. Linear versus curvilinear functions.* J. Amer. Geriat. Soc. 19:8, 721-728, August 1971.

2. Krall, L. P. *When is diabetes?* Med. Clin. N. America 49:4, 893-904, July 1965.

3. Schoen, A. W. *Automated multiphasic health testing programs directory,* 1971-1972, second edition. Burbank, Bioscience Publications, Inc.

4. Faludi, G., Bendersky, G., and Gerber, P. *Functional hypoglycemia in early latent diabetes.* Ann. New York Acad. Sc. 148:3, 868-874, 26 March 1968.

5. Waters, W. E., Withey, J. L., Kilpatrick, G. S., Wood, P. H. N., and Abernethy, M. *Ten-year haematological follow-up: mortality and haematological changes.* Brit. Med. J. 4:5686, 761-764, 27 December 1969.

6. Hammond, E. C. *Some preliminary findings on physical complaints from a prospective study of 1,064,004 men and women.* Amer. J. Public Health 54:1, 11-23, January 1964.

7. Weider, A., Mittelman, B., Wechsler, D., and Wolff, H. G. *Further developments of the Cornell Word Form.* Psychiat. Quart. 29:4, 588-594, October 1955.

8. Cheraskin, E. and Ringsdorf, W. M., Jr. *Resistance and susceptibility to oral disease. I. A study in gingivitis and carbohydrate metabolism.* J. Dent. Res. 44:2, 374-378, March-April 1965.

9. Cheraskin, E. and Ringsdorf, W. M., Jr. *Gingival state and carbohydrate metabolism.* J. Dent. Res. 44:3, 480-486, May-June 1965.

10. Cheraskin, E. and Ringsdorf, W. M., Jr. *Homeostasis: a study in carbohydrate metabolism.* J. Med. Assn. State Alabama 35:3, 173-182, September 1965.

11. Cheraskin, E. and Ringsdorf, W. M., Jr. *Tooth loss and carbohydrate metabolism.* New York State Dent. J. 31:8, 363-369, October 1965.

12. Cheraskin, E., Ringsdorf, W. M., Jr., Setyaadmadja, A. T. S. H., and Ginn, D. S. *Resistance and susceptibility to oral disease: III. A study in clinical tooth mobility and carbohydrate metabolism.* J. California Dent. Assn. 41:5, 416-420, October 1965.

13. Cheraskin, E., Ringsdorf, W. M., Jr., Setyaadmadja, A. T. S. H., and Ginn, D. S. *Resistance and susceptibility to oral disease: II. A study in periodontometry and carbohydrate metabolism.* Periodontics 3:6, 296-300, November-December 1965.

14. Cheraskin, E., Ringsdorf, W. M., Jr., Setyaadmadja, A. T. S. H., and Barrett, R. A. *Stomatology and the total organism: a study in carbohydrate metabolism.* Revista Ital. di Stomatol. 21:7, 651-667, 1966.

15. Cheraskin, E. and Ringsdorf, W. M., Jr. *Electrocardiographic standards of health: II. P wave duration [Lead I] in presumably healthy dental students.* J. Med. Assn. State Alabama 38:8, 708-711, February 1969.

16. Cheraskin, E. and Ringsdorf, W. M., Jr. *Electrocardiography and carbohydrate metabolism: I. P-wave length [Lead I] in presumably healthy young men.* J. Med. Assn. State Alabama 38:11, 1011-1014, May 1969.

17. Cheraskin, E. and Ringsdorf, W. M., Jr. *The edentulous patient. II. Xerostomia and the blood sugar level.* J. Amer. Geriat. Soc. 17:10, 966-968, October 1969.

18. Barrett, R. A., Cheraskin, E., and Ringsdorf, W. M., Jr. *Serum cholesterol as a predictor of capillaropathy.* Angiology 21:7, 462-467, July-August 1970.

Predictive Medicine

19. Ringsdorf, W. M., Jr., Cheraskin, E., and Hollis, C. F. *Levels of blood sugar and blood glucose in relation to systemic and oral health.* Dent. Progress 3:2, 121-124, January 1963.

20. Cheraskin, E. and Ringsdorf, W. M., Jr. *Gingival tenderness and carbohydrate metabolism.* Amer. J. Med. Sc. 246:6, 727-733, December 1963.

21. Cheraskin, E., Ringsdorf, W. M., Jr., and White, W. L., Jr. *Dry mouth and carbohydrate metabolism.* J. Amer. Geriat. Soc. 12:4, 337-344, April 1964.

22. Cheraskin, E. and Ringsdorf, W. M., Jr. *Furunculosis and carbohydrate metabolism.* J. Med. Assn. State Alabama 34:6, 153-157, December 1964.

23. Setyaadmadja, A. T. S. H., Cheraskin, E., and Ringsdorf, W. M., Jr. *Ascorbic acid and carbohydrate metabolism. I. The cortisone-glucose tolerance test.* J. Amer. Geriat. Soc. 13:10, 924-934, October 1965.

24. Cheraskin, E. and Ringsdorf, W. M., Jr. *Carbohydrate metabolism and carcinomatosis.* Cancer 17:2, 159-162, February 1964.

25. Cheraskin, E. and Ringsdorf, W. M., Jr. *Epilepsy and the cortisone-glucose tolerance test.* J. Lancet 83:6, 248-250, June 1963.

26. Stanton, G. *Diet and dental caries; the phosphate sequestration hypothesis.* New York State Dent. J. 35:7, 399-407, August-September 1969.

27. Dubos, R. J. *Mirage of health.* 1959. New York, Harper and Brothers. p. 100.

Physiologic Versus Normal Values

Epidemiology is the only way of asking some questions in medicine, one way of asking others [and no way at all to ask many].
— J. N. Morris.

Earlier chapters have outlined differences between conventional and predictive medicine. If one could single out one, if not the most, important distinction, it would center about the topic of *data interpretation.*

The term *normal* stems from the Latin *normalis,* which means according to the pattern. Hence, in its purest sense etymologically (and this is its statistical connotation), normal suggests the *typical,* the *usual,* the *average.*

The clinician, however, usually employs the word *normal* to define the *healthy* state. For example, he frequently remarks that a patient is normal or that the blood sugar or cholesterol values are normal. In fact, the word normal is used to describe the healthy state in every area of patient evaluation.

Hence, in the practitioner's mind, normal becomes interchangeable with that which is healthy. The simplest example that average, or normal, and healthy are not synonymous is the fact that 95 percent of Americans suffer with dental decay. It is, therefore, normal (meaning typical or usual) to have this problem. In other words, the average American has it. However, it is obviously not healthy or physiologic to exhibit dental caries.

Fundamentally, *three* techniques are employed to develop

61

standards for health and disease. This will be the subject of this chapter.[1]

The Epidemiologic Approach

The most common technique for determining the so-called normal value is to ascertain the parameter in question in a large sample of presumably well individuals.[2] Particular mention should be made that most criteria for health are generally quite arbitrary (e.g., ambulatory subjects, hospital personnel). The data are then arrayed and generally found to fit the typical unimodal or Gaussian curve. Then, on a purely arbitrary basis, the mean and two standard deviations (95 percent of the values) are held to represent the physiologic range for the parameter under consideration.

Typical of studies which fall in this category is one released by Bryan, Wearne, Viau, Musser, Schoonmaker, and Thiers.[3] In their own words, they indicate the composition of the group defined as healthy and the method of establishing the physiologic range. Table 6-1 shows the 95 percent limits of a normal population of students, employees,

Table 6-1
Normal Ranges (95% limits) and Expanded
Ranges Used for Criteria of Normality[3]

Determination	Normal range	Expanded range
Urea nitrogen [mg./100 ml.]	8-23	7-25
Glucose [mg./100 ml.]	75-110	65-120
Sodium [mEq/L.]	131-141	130-142
Potassium [mEq/L.]	3.6-4.8	3.5-4.9
Chloride [mEq/L.]	97-108	94-110
Carbon dioxide [mEq/L.]	26-35	24-37
Calcium [mg./100 ml.]	8.5-11.0	8.0-11.2
Phosphorus [mg./100 ml.]	2.5-4.5	2.0-4.9
Total protein [gm./100 ml.]	6.4-7.9	6.0-8.1
Albumin [gm./100 ml.]	3.5-5.0	3.1-5.2
Uric acid [mg./100 ml.]	2.0-7.5	0.0-8.5

health examinees, and blood bank donors as obtained in this laboratory for each of the 11 determinations.

Three points about table 6-1 deserve special consideration. First, the assumption is made that students, employees, health examinees, and blood bank donors are healthy. This hypothesis is not based upon fact. Actually, most multiple testing programs of such persons indicate that a significant number has one or more previously undetected diseases. For example, according to the United States Department of Health, Education, and Welfare,[4] the incidence of one or more chronic conditions (illnesses, diseases, or impairments) even in young people less than 17 years old was one in five (20.1 percent) in 1962-1963 and has climbed to almost one in four (23.2 percent) in 1966-1967 (figure 6.1). Hence, one must recognize that the criteria for health sampling are very arbitrary. Second, a range of two standard deviations is

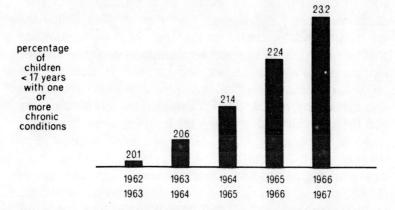

United States Department of Health, Education and Welfare. National Center for Health Statistics. Series 10, Numbers 5 13, 25, 37 and 43. January 1964 – January 1968. Current Estiments from the Health Interview Survey. Superintendent of Documents. United States Government Printing Office. Washington, D.C.

Figure 6-1. The percentage of children under 17 years of age in the civilian, noninstitutionalized population with one or more chronic conditions.

utilized for describing the physiologic (healthy) limits. Multiphasic screening of allegedly healthy persons indicates that one cannot make the assumption that two standard deviations (which include 95 percent of the population) are well. Thus, we must appreciate the arbitrariness of these limits. Finally, the authors, quite categorically, expand the range without any explanation (table 6-1): "It also shows a set of slightly expanded ranges which were employed as criteria of clinical normality and abnormality for this experiment."[3]

It should be abundantly evident from this brief discussion that the presently employed method for ascertaining the physiologic (so-called normal) range for a diagnostic parameter is most arbitrary.[5-9]

The Sta-ten Concept

For the reasons offered earlier, many investigators have been concerned with the development of more meaningful standards for health and disease. Casey et al.[10-12] divide the typical unimodal pattern into sta-tens which are ten units of standard deviation. The mode, according to these authors, represents the ideal and is assigned a score of 5. Values which fall 0-0.5 standard deviation below the mode are numbered 4 and called low modal, 0.5-1.0 standard deviation below are numbered 3 (mild decrease), 1.0-1.5 below are assigned 2 (moderate decrease), 1.5-2.0 below are listed as 1 (marked decrease), and 2.0 and below are numbered 0 and represent very marked decrease. In conventional medicine only values outside of two standard deviations are viewed as pathologic. Similarly, the values 6, 7, 8, 9, and 10 are utilized for scores above the mode in one-half standard deviation groups.

The most obvious benefit from this system is its recognition that small variations from the mode signify the development of a pathologic process. The most apparent shortcoming of this approach is the assumption that the mode is synonymous with optimal health.

The Symptom-sign-free Concept

From the earlier discussion it is clear that there is still considerable debate as to what should be regarded as the *physiologic* limits for a particular biochemical parameter. The point has been made that the present concept of a physiologic range is developed from an analysis of *presumably* healthy subjects. Even though such persons are not obviously ill, they may, nonetheless, have an undetected disorder or exhibit subtle symptoms and signs which are clearly not suggestive of a state of health (chapter 4).

It seems fair to assume that an individual *without* symptoms and signs is probably healthier than one *with* clinical findings.[13] Considering this assumption, a study is here reported of the fasting blood glucose range in groups with and without symptoms and signs.[14]

One hundred dental patients, seen for routine care, were questioned regarding symptoms and examined for signs generally recognized as indicative of diabetes mellitus. Though the main emphasis was placed upon the oral cavity, some few extraoral symptoms (polyphagia, polydipsia, and polyuria) were also recorded. Each individual was also studied by means of the glucose tolerance test as described by Mosenthal and Barry.[15] For purposes of this report, only the fasting blood glucose determinations will be considered.

An analysis of fasting blood glucose was first made for those of the original 100 subjects free of a *single* extraoral symptom. The 82 subjects without polyphagia (though some may have had polyuria and/or polydipsia) showed a mean and standard deviation of 81±21 mg. percent. A similar analysis of the 82 polydipsia-free patients (though some may have reported polyphagia and/or polyuria) yielded values of 81±20 mg. percent. Finally, the 71 patients without polyuria (with or without polyphagia and/or polydipsia) netted a score of 80±18 mg. percent. It is clear from an analysis of those patients lacking any one of these findings that the

no extraoral symptoms
(no polyphagia, polyuria, polydipsia)

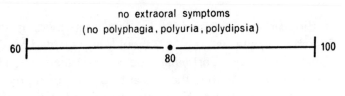

60 |————————•————————| 100
80

no gingival pathosis

67 |————————•———————| 89
78

no oral symptoms
(no dry & burning mouth, gingival tenderness)

71 |————•————| 85
78

no dental stigmata
(full dental complement, no clinical tooth mobility)

68 |————•————| 84
76

no oral roentgenographic pathosis
(no alveolar bone loss, no periodontal widening)

70 |———•———| 82
76

no dental stigmata
no oral roentgenographic pathosis

72 |—•—| 76
74

no oral symptoms
no dental stigmata
no oral roentgenographic pathosis

74 |•| 76
75

Figure 6-2. The technique for the development of the physiologic range for fasting blood glucose by developing a progressively symptomless and sign-free group. By this method, the range progressively shrinks.

means and standard deviations are very similar. In order to develop a simple chart, figure 6-2 shows only the mean and standard deviation for the 50 subjects *without* the extraoral symptoms of polyphagia, polyuria, *and* polydipsia (80±20 mg. percent).

In order to establish the fasting blood glucose range on a more quantitatable basis, gingival health was studied. Sixteen of the original 100 subjects demonstrated physiologic gingival hue, color, stippling, and sulci around the teeth. It is important to emphasize that some of these patients may have reported one or more of the extraoral symptoms previously mentioned. This group, characterized by healthy gingiva, showed a value of 78±11 mg. percent (figure 6-2). Compared to the initial analysis, the mean has decreased from 80 to 78, and the standard deviation has been cut in half (from 20 to 11).

Similar analyses were made for the 38 subjects without oral symptoms (gingival tenderness, dry and burning mouth), for the 16 subjects with no dental stigmata (full complement of teeth and no clinical tooth mobility), and for the 11 persons without oral roentgenographic evidence of disease (no alveolar bone loss and no periodontal widening). All of these values are depicted in figure 6-2.

Finally, the means and standard deviations were derived for the groups of subjects without *combinations* of symptoms and signs. Figure 6-2 shows the scores for the five patients without dental stigmata *and* oral roentgenographic pathosis. Also shown (at the very bottom) are the values for the three subjects without oral symptoms, dental signs or X-ray evidence of pathosis.

A number of points are worthy of mention. First, two thirds of the asymptomatic patients, in terms of extraoral findings, range from 60 to 100 mg. percent fasting blood glucose. Interestingly enough, this is the presently accepted range.[15] Second, by employing different criteria for physiologic state, the means decrease slightly and the ranges shrink dramatically. Third, by stiffening the requirements for health (the insistence of progressively fewer symptoms and signs), the range shrinks to almost zero. This technique for the establishment of physiologic ranges has been investigated for a number of different parameters.[16-18]

The development of physiologic standards by means of this technique can be accomplished in many ways. Described here is one example from a study of 328 presumably healthy dentists and their wives.[1]

Each subject completed the Cornell Medical Index Health Questionnaire, and the total number of affirmative responses (suggestive of pathosis) was recorded. Additionally, a non-fasting serum cholesterol determination was made.

Figure 6-3 shows (on the abscissa) the age groups. Pictured

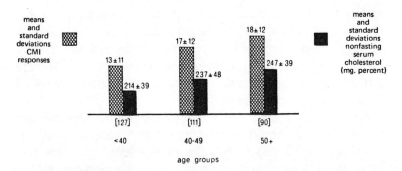

Figure 6-3. The relationship of age (on the abscissa) to clinical symptoms and signs as judged by the Cornell Medical Index Health Questionnaire (stippled bars) and nonfasting serum cholesterol (black columns). The data confirm the well-established observation that, with advancing age, symptoms and signs and serum cholesterol increase.

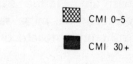

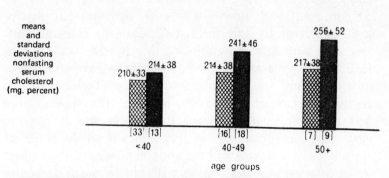

Figure 6-4. The relationship of age (on the horizontal axis) with serum cholesterol in relatively healthy (stippled columns) and sick (black bar) groups of people. In the latter, the serum cholesterol rises with time; in the former there is no significant change. This suggests a physiologic range for serum cholesterol.

on the ordinate (stippled columns) are the number of positive responses on the questionnaire. The chart confirms the well-established clinical observation that, with time, people show progressively more symptoms and signs. Figure 6-3 also confirms the well-known observation that, with time (black columns), the serum cholesterol rises. Figure 6-4 pictorially portrays three groups in terms of age (horizontal axis). The black bars represent subjects with 30 or more positive responses on the Cornell Medical Index Health Questionnaire. The evidence indicates a rapid rise in serum cholesterol (214 to 241 to 256) with advancing age. In sharp contrast, in the group showing only 0-5 positive responses (stippled columns), the nonfasting serum cholesterol remains strikingly constant (210 to 217) with time. On the assumption that the latter group is healthier, then the mean serum cholesterol derived from this group should be regarded as more physiologic.

Mention should be made that, by this technique, the serum cholesterol range is more restricted than is generally held to be consistent with health. Moreover, derivation of physiologic standards by this technique begins to compare very favorably with some new thinking in this area. According to R. E. Hodges: "If we assume that *average* levels of cholesterol in the serum are equivalent to *normal* levels, then the textbook figure of 150 to 250 mg. per 100 ml. would be acceptable for most Americans. But if we accept the realistic view that *Americans are in the midst of an epidemic of coronary heart disease* and that this epidemic results, at least in large measure, from abnormally high levels of serum cholesterol, then we must reexamine our definition of "normal". The Framingham studies and others have shown that there is a continuing influence of serum cholesterol concentrations, from very low to very high, on the prevalence of coronary heart disease. If we were to pick an arbitrary point on the curve below which most cases of coronary heart disease could be avoided, we might select 220 mg. per 100 ml. Above this level, the prevalence of coronary disease rises rapidly."[19]

Summary

At the present time, standards for health and disease can be derived by *three* different methods. The first is based upon the assumption that 95 percent of the population is healthy. This is, admittedly, a highly arbitrary method. A second, less arbitrary, technique employs the hypothesis that the farther away from the mode for a particular parameter, the greater the possibility of pathosis. The final method, still less arbitrary, is based upon the thesis that standards for health should parallel the relatively symptomless and signfree clinical pattern. Additional support for this concept has been underlined most lucidly by Casey as follows:

"Standard deviations were developed over 50 years ago as yardsticks of variation on either side of the mean or average. Usually two standard deviations on either side of the mean contain 97 percent of the observations. This is the dividing line between normal and abnormal in most laboratory and clinical textbooks. Generally, florid or far-advanced clinical disease is characterized by a greater standard deviation, including uremia, anasarca, coronary thrombosis, diabetic coma, stroke, which represent extreme and often terminal disease."

"A sophisticated history and physical examination will often disclose signs and symptoms beginning with 1.5 standard deviations above or below the mean, and clinical disease is often proven by appropriate laboratory tests."[1][2]

References

1. Cheraskin, E. and Ringsdorf, W. M., Jr. *Predictive medicine: VI. Physiologic versus normal values.* J. Amer. Geriat. Soc. 19:8, 729-736, August 1971.

2. Ivy, A. C. *What is normal or normality?* Quart. Bull. Northwestern Univ. 18:1, 22-32, Spring Quarter 1944.

3. Bryan, D. J., Wearne, J. L., Viau, A., Musser, A. W., Schoonmaker, F. W., and Thiers, R. E. *Profile of admission chemical data by multichannel automation: an evaluative experiment.* Clin. Chem. 12:3, 137-143, March 1966.

4. United States Department of Health, Education, and Welfare. National Center for Health Statistics. *Current estimates from the Health Interview Survey.* Series 10:5, 13, 25, 37, and 43. January 1964-January 1968. Washington, D. C., Superintendent of Documents, United States Government Printing Office.

5. Ratner, H. *Practical difficulties in defining the word "normal" in medicine.* Illinois Med. J. 97:3, 143-145, March 1950.

6. Mainland, D. *Normal values in medicine.* Ann. New York Acad. Sc. 161:2, 527-537, 30 September 1969.

7. Sunderman, F. W., Jr. *Computer applications in laboratory medicine: the delineation of normal values.* Ann. New York Acad. Sc. 161:2, 549-571, 30 September 1969.

8. Orfanakis, N. G., Ostlund, R. E., Bishop, C. R., and Athens, J. W. *Normal blood leukocyte concentration values.* Amer. J. Clin. Path. 53:5, 647-651, May 1970.

9. Simonson, E. *Differentiation between normal and abnormal in electro-cardiography.* 1961. St. Louis, The C. V. Mosby Company.

10. Casey, A. E., Downey, E. L., Elliott, C. B., Lohmann, H. J., and Meigs, L.

Predictive Medicine

C. *The role of the pathologist in the completely automated laboratory.* Alabama J. Med. Sc. 4:2, 145-150, April 1967.

11. Gilbert, F. E., Casey, A. E., Downey, E. L., Thomason, S., and Deacy, J. V. *Admission inorganic phosphorus correlated with discharge diagnosis and other metabolic profile components.* Alabama J. Med. Sc. 7:3, 343-349, July 1970.

12. Casey, A. E. and Downey, E. *Further use of sta-tens in the recording, reporting, analysis, and retrieval of automated computerized laboratory and clinical data.* Amer. J. Clin. Path. 53:5, 748-754, May 1970.

13. Engel, G. L. *A unified concept of health and disease.* Persp. Biol. Med. 3:4, 459-485, Summer 1960.

14. Cheraskin, E. and Ringsdorf, W. M., Jr. *Physiologic fasting blood glucose: range or point?* J. Dent. Med. 16:2, 96-98, April 1961.

15. Mosenthal, H. O. and Barry, E. *Criteria for and interpretation of normal glucose tolerance test.* Ann. Int. Med. 33:5, 1175-1194, November 1950.

16. Ringsdorf, W. M., Jr., Cheraskin, E., and Hollis, C. F. *Biochemical standards of health: II. Leukocyte count.* J. Tennessee St. Dent. Assn. 43:2, 126-133, April 1963.

17. Ringsdorf, W. M., Jr. and Cheraskin, E. *Biochemical standards of health: III. Fasting blood glucose.* New York J. Dent. 33:5, 185-187, May 1963.

18. Cheraskin, E., Ringsdorf, W. M., Jr., Setyaadmadja, A. T. S. H., and Barrett, R. A. *Biochemical standards of health: IV. Three-hour oral glucose tolerance test.* Acta Diabet. Latina 4:3, 386-396, July-September 1967.

19. Hodges, R. E. *Dietary and other factors which influence serum lipids.* J. Amer. Dietet. Assn. 52:3, 198-201, March 1968.

The Specificity of Tests

A new scientific truth does not triumph by convincing its opponents and making them see the light; but, rather, because its opponents eventually die and a new generation grows up that is familiar with it.　　　　　　—Max Planck

Earlier chapters have developed the philosophy of predictive medicine and described some of the unique features that set it apart from traditional medicine. This chapter considers whether specific testing procedures are pathognomonic (distinctly characteristic) of a particular disease.[1] For example, the glucose tolerance test is usually regarded as a detector of diabetes mellitus and the uric acid level as a specific indicator of gout.

In chapter 4 the point was made that clinical disease usually begins with several seemingly unrelated and nonspecific symptoms and signs. With time, the clinical findings increase in number and begin to localize in systems, organs, and tissues. Finally, as more time lapses (months, years, or even decades), the constellation satisfies the textbook definition of a particular disease. Therefore, one of the problems in assigning a pathognomonic role to a particular test is that there is usually an arbitrary definition of what constitutes a particular disease syndrome.

The picture is further complicated by the fact that just about every test which has been studied has been shown to be related to many different disorders. One explanation for this is that most of the prevalent chronic diseases are complex metabolic dysfunctions that affect many systems, organs, and tissues. For example, a decrease in glucose

7

tolerance is characteristic of a score of diverse and allegedly nondiabetic syndromes (table 7-1).[2] Recent evidence[3-4] has disclosed numerous biochemical parallelisms. For example,[4] subjects with low inorganic phosphorus also show low calcium, uric acid, potassium, total protein, and beta globulin. In other cases subjects with low inorganic phosphorus show regularly high carbon dioxide, creatine phosphokinase, cephalin flocculation, bilirubin, and blood sugar. Hence, it seems more tenable that abnormal biochemical test findings in the early ill-defined incubation stages of disease are more likely a measure of the *syndrome of sickness* rather than a manifestation of a specific, sharply defined disorder.

Table 7-1
Clinical Conditions Which May Exhibit
a Reduction in Glucose Tolerance

Psychologic disorders
Cancer
Hypertension
Hyperlipemia
Atherosclerosis and arteriosclerosis
Coronary heart disease
Obesity
Gout
Pregnancy
Congenital malformations or anomalies
Sterility
Drug suppression of ovulation
Eye disorders
Skin disorders
Infectious disorders
Multiple sclerosis
Peptic ulcer
Renal failure
Liver disease
Hyperthyroidism
Osteoporosis
Pulmonary emphysema
Tic douloureux
Aging

Two examples will be used to demonstrate this concept: (1) serum uric acid and nongout problems, and (2) serum triglycerides and noncardiac syndromes.

Serum Uric Acid and Nongout Problems

Mention was made earlier that hyperuricemia is usually regarded in most circles as pathognomonic of gout. The additional point has been made (chapter 2) that uric acid may be considered as one parameter in the coronary proneness profile. Finally, it should be underlined that uric acid is the fourth most commonly employed biochemical test in multiphasic screening programs.[5] To emphasize the nonspecificity of this particular biochemical parameter, figure 7-1 shows the relationship of serum uric acid (on the abscissa) and mean height of the P wave in Lead I (on the ordinate) in 72 presumably healthy subjects.[1] First, it is important to note that the relationship is parabolic rather than linear. Thus, the highest and presumably the most abnormal P_1 values (stippled columns) parallel relative hypo- *and* hyperuricemia. The smallest and probably the most physiologic electrocardiographic values (black bar) are found with serum uric acid levels of 4-5 mg. percent. This is consistent with earlier observations (chapter 5) showing curvilinear rather than linear parallelisms. Second, the relationship between serum uric acid and mean height of P_1 suggests that hyperuricemia is not exclusively associated with what is usually regarded as the classical picture of gout. This is additionally confirmed from a study of 200 patients with hyperuricemia.[6] The most common causes of urate elevation were azotemia (20 percent), acidosis (20 percent), and ingestion of diuretics (20 percent). Only 12 percent had a history of gout.

To demonstrate further the nonspecific concept, figure 7-2 pictures serum uric acid on the horizontal axis and psychologic scores (as judged by the Cornell Word Form-2 test) on the vertical axis in the same 72 presumably healthy subjects.[1]

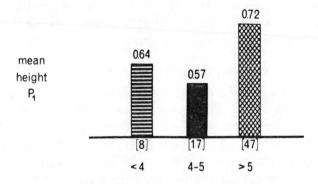

Figure 7-1. The relationship of serum uric acid (on the abscissa) and the height of P_1 (on the ordinate). The highest, and presumably the most pathologic P_1 heights are noted with relative hyper- and hypouricemia. The lowest and probably the most physiologic P_1 height (black column) is found in the middle range of serum uric acid. It is noteworthy that there is such a parallelism between serum uric acid and an allegedly nongout finding. This underlines the nonspecific nature of serum uric acid.

The earlier two conclusions obtain here. First, the relationship is curvilinear rather than linear. As a matter of fact, the highest (and supposedly most pathologic psychic mean score) occurs in the group with hypouricemia. Second, here is another expression of the diagnostic nonspecific nature of serum uric acid, since psychologic imbalance is generally not held to be part of the gout syndrome.

Serum Triglycerides and Noncardiac Syndromes

At the present time, major concern is being directed to the coronary proneness profile (chapter 2). Biochemically, serum cholesterol and serum triglycerides are recognized as predictors of coronary artery disease. The implication is that these two barometers of lipid metabolism are exclusively

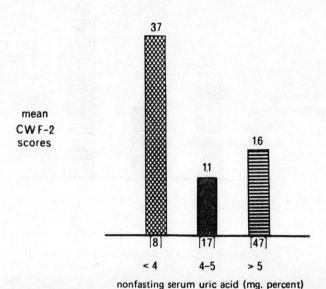

Figure 7-2. The relationship of serum uric acid (on the horizontal axis) and psychologic scores as judged by the Cornell Word Form-2 test (on the vertical axis). The highest, and presumably the most pathologic, CWF-2 scores are noted with relative hyper- and hypouricemia. The lowest and probably the most physiologic CWF-2 score (black columns) is found in the middle range of serum uric acid. It is interesting that there is such a relationship between serum uric acid and an allegedly nongout finding. This underscores the nonspecific nature of serum uric acid.

involved in cardiovascular disease. To underscore that this is not true, two observations are reported here.[1]

Nonfasting serum triglyceride levels and the frequency of reported gastrointestinal findings in 100 apparently healthy individuals were compared (figure 7-3). Shown on the x-axis are the serum triglyceride group and on the y-axis the mean number of reported gastrointestinal symptoms and signs. It is noteworthy that the relationship is parabolic with the

77

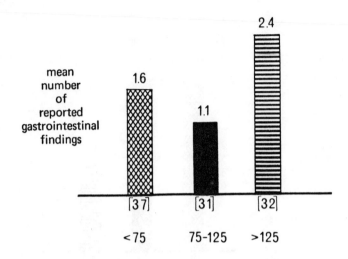

nonfasting serum triglycerides (mg. percent)

Figure 7-3. The relationship of serum triglycerides (on the abscissa) and the mean number of reported gastrointestinal findings (on the ordinate). The greatest numbers of gastrointestinal findings are noted with relative hyper- and hypotriglyceridemia. The lowest and most physiologic gastrointestinal finding (black column) is found in the middle range of serum triglycerides. It is noteworthy that there is such a parallelism between serum triglycerides and an allegedly noncardiac finding. This underlines the nonspecific nature of serum triglycerides.

greatest mean gastrointestinal scores (stippled bars) characterized by *both* hyper- and hypotriglyceridemia. Although the interrelationship is not explicable, this data suggests that serum triglyceride levels may be useful in the early detection of gastroenteric problems.

Figure 7-4 relates serum triglycerides to the seemingly unrelated reporting of respiratory symptoms and signs in the same group of 100 persons.[1] The findings with serum triglycerides and respiratory symptoms and signs are similar to those observed with serum triglycerides and gastrointestinal findings and with serum uric acid and both psychologic scores and electrocardiography.

Even among the relatively classical disease states it has been noted that hypertriglyceridemia is a feature of gout, diabetes mellitus, atherosclerosis, and obesity. Says W. K. Ishmael: "The association between impaired carbohydrate metabolism and atherosclerosis, and between dietary carbohydrate [sucrose] and hypertriglyceridemia, and the in-

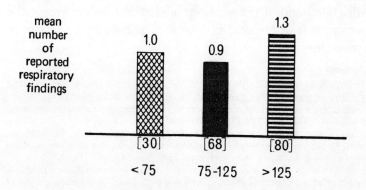

nonfasting serum triglycerides (mg. percent)

Figure 7-4. The relationship of serum triglycerides (on the abscissa) and the mean number of reported respiratory findings (on the ordinate). The greatest numbers of respiratory findings are noted with relative hyper- and hypotriglyceridemia. The lowest and most physiologic respiratory findings (black column) are found in the middle range of serum triglycerides. It is noteworthy that there is such a parallelism between serum triglycerides and an allegedly noncardiac finding. This underlines the nonspecific nature of serum triglycerides.

creased triglyceride concentration accompanying hyper-uricemia, are consistent with the hypothesis that the genetically associated diseases of gout, diabetes, atherosclerosis, and obesity are causally related to carbohydrate [sucrose] induced or aggravated hypertriglyceridemia."[7]

Summary

In the classical stages of disease various biochemical tests may be highly diagnostic. However, in the *early* development of disease these tests are not pathognomonic or specific for a particular disease syndrome. Rather, biochemical testing, for predictive purposes, must be regarded as a measure of the *syndrome of sickness*. This reflects the health status of the entire body and, if the warnings are heeded, will intercept the development of classical disease in a specific tissue, organ, or system site.

References

1. Cheraskin, E. and Ringsdorf, W. M., Jr. *Predictive medicine: VII. The specificity of tests.* J. Amer. Geriat. Soc. 19:9, 802-806, September 1971.

2. Cheraskin, E. and Ringsdorf, W. M., Jr. *Diabetic dilemma in dentistry.* Acta Diabet. Latina 8:2, 228-277, March-April 1971.

3. Gertler, M. M., Leetma, H. E., Saluste, E., Welsh, J. J., Rusk, H. A., Covalt, D. A., and Rosenberger, J. *Carbohydrate, insulin, and lipid interrelationship in ischemic vascular disease.* Geriatrics 25:5, 134-148, May, 1970.

4. Gilbert, F. E., Casey, A. E., Downey, E. L., Thomason, S., and Deacy, J. V. *Admission inorganic phosphorus correlated with discharge diagnoses and other metabolic profile components.* Alabama J. Med. Sc. 7:3, 343-349, July 1970.

5. Schoen, A. W. *Automated multiphasic health testing programs directory,* 1971-1972, second edition. Burbank, Bioscience Publications, Inc.

6. Paulus, H. E., Coutts, A., Calabro, J. J., and Klinenberg, J. R. *Clinical significance of hyperuricemia in routinely screened hospitalized men.* J. A. M. A. 211:2, 277-281, 12 January 1970.

7. Ishmael, W. K. *Atherosclerotic vascular disease in familial gout, diabetes and obesity.* Med. Times 94:12, 157-162, February 1966.

Familial Versus Genetic Factors

People love genetics as an explantion for disease. If a disease is said to be genetic, you don't have to do anything about it. However, if a disease has an environmental cause, the individual, whether patient or clinician, has a responsibility for making the change or changes to eliminate or control the disease.
—Denis P. Burkitt.

Except for a comparatively few hereditary diseases, life experiences, rather than inherited characteristics, may be the major factors that make one individual significantly different from the next.[1] Thus, more attention must be directed to environmental forces in the genesis of disease. This approach minimizes the element of hopelessness which frequently follows when diseases are ascribed to purely hereditary factors.

This chapter is designed to demonstrate another unique feature of a predictive medicine program. Specifically, an attempt will be made to underline environmental influences in a number of diagnostic areas usually not regarded as related to the environment.[2] Thus, environmental effects upon dietary intake, blood enzymes, blood biochemical patterns, and clinical signs and symptoms will be investigated.

Diet and Environment

The importance of diet in predictive medicine will be dealt with in some detail in chapters 9, 11, 14. For the present, it is relevant to examine the diet as it relates to the environment.

Daily refined carbohydrate consumption was established from a seven-day dietary survey in a group of 82 dentists, their 82 wives, and in 82 wives of other dentists age-paired with the wives of the dentists in this study.[3] This included such foods as table sugar, desserts, sweet beverages, and bakery items. Table 8-1 shows that a statistically significant correlation (r = +0.520, P <0.01) for daily refined carbohydrate consumption exists only between the husband and wife. Additionally, an analysis was made of the younger and older couples (table 8-1). Since the correlation coefficient is higher (r = +0.669) in the older couples, it is reasonable to conclude that, with advancing age, couples tend to eat more alike with regard to refined carbohydrate foods (figure 8-1). Essentially, the findings are similar with total carbohydrates,[3] total calories,[4] fats,[5] proteins,[6] and vitamin A consumption.[7]

Table 8-1
Correlation Coefficients for Daily
Refined Carbohydrate Consumption

	Number of pairs	r	P
Husband vs wife	82	+0.520	<0.01*
Husband vs unrelated female	82	+0.002	>0.05
Wife vs unrelated female	82	-0.078	>0.05
Husband vs wife			
[husband's age <41]	40	+0.442	<0.01*
[husband's age 41+]	42	+0.669	<0.01*
Husband vs unrelated female			
[husband's age <41]	40	+0.109	>0.05
[husband's age 41+]	42	-0.094	>0.05
Wife vs unrelated female			
[age <40]	43	-0.105	>0.05
[age 40+]	39	-0.015	>0.05

*Statistically significant correlation coefficient.

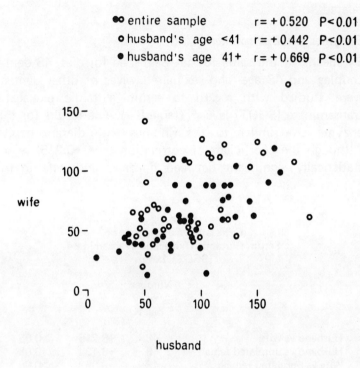

Figure 8-1. The relationship of daily refined carbohydrate consumption (in grams) in the husband (on the abscissa) and in the wife (on the ordinate). For the entire sample, the correlation coefficient (r = +0.520) is highly significant (P <0.01). The correlation coefficient (r = +0.669, P <0.01) is even higher in the older married couples (black dots).

It is clear from these limited observations that environmental influences must play a significant role in dietary patterns, since the average married couple is not genetically related.

Enzymes and Environment

By means of the same format described for diet, 48 dental couples and 48 age- and sex-paired wives of other dentists were studied with regard to serum glutamic oxalacetic transaminase (SGOT) levels[8] (table 8-2). The results for this enzyme are similar to the findings with dietary habits. Although the coefficient of correlation (r = +0.215) is not statistically significant between husband and wife in the

Table 8-2
Correlation Coefficients of
Serum Glutamic Oxalacetic Transaminase
[SGOT] Levels

	Number of pairs	r	P
Husband vs wife	48	+0.215	>0.05
Husband vs unrelated female	48	+0.132	>0.05
Wife vs unrelated female	48	-0.050	>0.05
Husband vs wife			
[husband's age <44]	25	-0.023	>0.05
[husband's age 44+]	23	+0.686	<0.01*
Husband vs unrelated female			
[husband's age <44]	25	+0.258	>0.05
[husband's age 44+]	23	-0.058	>0.05
Wife vs unrelated female			
[age <43]	22	-0.071	>0.05
[age 43+]	26	-0.123	>0.05

*Statistically significant correlation coefficient.

whole group, it increases to a highly significant value in the older couples (r = +0.686, P <0.01). Thus, the longer these couples were together, the more similar were their SGOT levels (figure 8-2). Similar findings have been noted for lactic dehydrogenase (LDH)[9] with correlation coefficients reaching +0.937 (P <0.01) for the married couples.

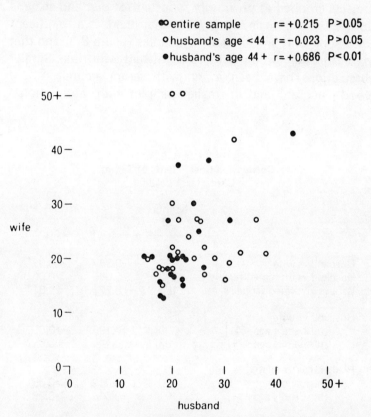

∞ entire sample   r = +0.215   P>0.05
○ husband's age <44   r = −0.023   P>0.05
● husband's age 44 +   r = +0.686   P<0.01

wife

husband

Figure 8-2. The relationship of serum glutamic oxalacetic transaminase [SGOT] in the husband (on the horizontal axis) and in the wife (on the vertical axis). For the entire sample, the correlation (r = +0.215) is not significant (P >0.05). The correlation coefficients for the younger (open circles) and older (black dots) couples are markedly different. A statistically significant correlation coefficient (r = +0.686, P <0.01) is noted in the older married group.

The conclusion may be drawn from these data that environmental factors influence enzyme levels, since genetic variables do not play a significant role in married couples.

Biochemistry and Environment

Table 8-3 summarizes the results for serum cholesterol in 588 subjects grouped as previously reported for diet and enzyme studies.[2] Once again, it is clear that there is a significant correlation only in the married couples (figure 8-3) and that the correlation becomes more significant with time. Similar observations have been found with serum albumin[10] and blood glucose[11] and in smaller samples with serum choles-

Table 8-3
Correlation Coefficients of Serum
Cholesterol Levels

	Number of pairs	r	P
Husband vs wife	196	+0.367	<0.01*
Husband vs unrelated female	196	+0.085	>0.05
Wife vs unrelated female	196	+0.271	<0.01*
Husband vs wife			
[husband's age <41]	99	+0.196	>0.05
[husband's age 41+]	97	+0.440	<0.01*
Husband vs unrelated female			
[husband's age <41]	99	+0.012	>0.05
[husband's age 41+]	97	+0.016	>0.05
Wife vs unrelated female			
[age <39]	96	+0.129	>0.05
[age 39+]	100	+0.209	<0.05*

*Statistically significant correlation coefficient.

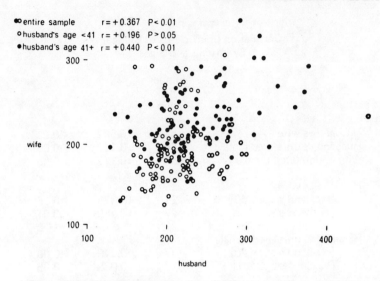

Figure 8-3. The relationship of nonfasting serum cholesterol (mg. percent) in the husband (on the horizontal axis) and in the wife (on the vertical axis). For the entire sample, the correlation coefficient (r = +0.367) is significant (P <0.01). The correlation coefficient (r = +0.440, P <0.01) is even higher in the older married couples (black dots).

terol.[12] Here is additional evidence, in the biochemical sphere, of the effect of the environment.

Clinical State and the Environment

Environmental effects may also be noted at the clinical level. Fifty-four dental couples and 54 age- and sex-paired wives of other dentists were studied in terms of clinical scores as determined by the Cornell Medical Index Health Questionnaire (CMI).[13] Table 8-4 outlines the relationships. The pattern is very similar to that earlier described at the dietary, enzymic, and biochemical levels. Specifically, there is a statistically significant correlation only in the married couples and the correlation increases with age (figure 8-4).

87

Table 8-4
Correlation Coefficients of Clinical
Symptoms and Signs

	Number of pairs	r	P
Husband vs wife	54	+0.522	<0.01*
Husband vs unrelated female	54	+0.122	>0.05
Wife vs unrelated female	54	+0.117	>0.05
Husband vs wife			
[husband's age <40]	27	+0.373	>0.05
[husband's age 40+]	27	+0.689	<0.01*
Husband vs unrelated female			
[husband's age <40]	27	+0.249	>0.05
[husband's age 40+]	27	-0.038	>0.05
Wife vs unrelated female			
[age <40]	35	+0.186	>0.05
[age 40+]	19	-0.247	>0.05

*Statistically significant correlation coefficient.

Additionally, these clinical parallelisms have been previously noted with overall symptoms and signs in a larger group[14] and with psychic findings.[15] In a recent random sample of 499 families, parents and children were compared for health and personality factors. Poor health in one parent was generally found to be associated with poor health in the other parent.[16]

Summary

There is no question but that genetic factors influence health and disease. However, it seems likely that genetic variables are not as overriding as previously held. Also, it is possible that there are environmental factors which can mask or trigger genetic problems. Finally, there is reasonable evidence

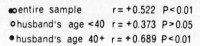

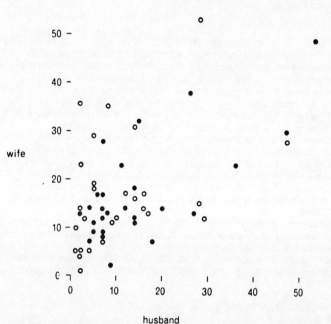

Figure 8-4. The relationship of the frequency of reported clinical symptoms and signs (CMI scores) in the husband (on the x-axis) and in the wife (on the y-axis). For the entire group, the correlation coefficients (r = +0.522) is significant (P <0.01). The correlation coefficient (r = +0.689, P <0.01) is even higher in the older married couples (black dots).

that the environment plays a role in diet, enzymes, bio-chemical state, and in the clinical picture. This is borne out by the fact that statistically significant correlations are noted in married couples who are not genetically linked. Over several generations these strong interrelationships have been observed to influence genetic transmission.

The most important item is the fact that more emphasis on

environmental factors is another unique feature of a predictive medicine program. In the final analysis, while it may be difficult to alter the environment, it is still easier than modifying genes.

References

1. Knobloch, H. and Pasamanick, B. *Seasonal variation in the births of the mentally deficient.* Amer. J. Pub. Health 48:9, 1201-1208, September 1958.

2. Cheraskin, E. and Ringsdorf, W. M., Jr. *Predictive medicine: VIII. Familial versus genetic factors.* J. Amer. Geriat. Soc. 19:10, 887-893, October 1971.

3. Cheraskin, E. and Ringsdorf, W. M., Jr. *Familial dietary patterns: II. Daily carbohydrate consumption.* J. Appl. Nutrit. 22:1 & 2, 17-22, Spring 1970.

4. Cheraskin, E. and Ringsdorf, W. M., Jr. *Familial dietary patterns: I. Daily caloric consumption.* J. Appl. Nutrit. 21:3 & 4, 70-73, Winter 1969.

5. Cheraskin, E. and Ringsdorf, W. M., Jr. *Familial dietary patterns: III. Daily fat consumption.* J. Appl. Nutrit. 22:3 & 4, 68-72, Fall-Winter 1970.

6. Cheraskin, E. and Ringsdorf, W. M., Jr. *Familial dietary patterns: IV. Daily protein consumption.* J. Appl. Nutrit. 23:1 & 2, 27-33, Spring 1971.

7. Cheraskin, E. and Ringsdorf, W. M., Jr. *Familial dietary patterns: Daily vitamin A consumption in the dentist and his wife.* Internat. J. Vit. Res. 40:2, 125-130, 1970.

8. Cheraskin, E. and Ringsdorf, W. M., Jr. *Familial enzymic patterns: I. Serum glutamic oxalacetic transaminase (SGOT) in the dentist and his wife.* Nutr. Rep. Internat. 1:2, 119-124, February 1970.

9. Cheraskin, E. and Ringsdorf, W. M., Jr. *Familial enzymic patterns: II. Lactic dehydrogenase (LDH) in the dentist and his wife.* Nutr. Rep. Internat. 1:2, 125-130, February 1970.

10. Cheraskin, E. and Ringsdorf, W. M., Jr. *Familial biochemical patterns: II. Serum albumin levels in the dentist and his wife.* Nutr. Rep. Internat. 1:5, 313-318, May 1970.

11. Cheraskin, E., Ringsdorf, W. M., Jr., Setyaadmadja, A. T. S. H., Barrett, R. A., Sibley, G. T., and Reid, R. W. *Environmental factors in blood glucose regulation.* J. Amer. Geriat. Soc. 16:7, 823-825, July 1968.

12. Cheraskin, E. and Ringsdorf, W. M., Jr. *Familial biochemical patterns: I. Serum cholesterol in the dentist and his wife.* J. Atheroscl. Res. 11:2, 247-250, May 1970.

13. Cheraskin, E. and Ringsdorf, W. M., Jr. *Frequency of reported symptoms and signs in the dentist and his wife.* Geriatrics 23:11, 158-160, November 1968.

14. Cheraskin, E. and Ringsdorf, W. M., Jr. *Familial clinical patterns: I. Reported symptoms and signs in the dentist and his wife.* Geriatrics 25:2, 123-126, February 1970.

15. Cheraskin, E. and Ringsdorf, W. M., Jr. *Familial factors in psychic adjustment.* J. Amer. Geriat. Soc. 17:6, 609-611, June 1969.

16. Hare, E. H. and Shaw, G. K. *A study in family health. II. A comparison of the health of fathers, mothers and children.* Brit. J. Psychiat. 111:475, 467-471, June 1965.

Diet

Our studies at Harvard among residents suggest that the average physician knows a little more about nutrition than the average secretary—unless the secretary has a weight problem, and then she probably knows more than the average physician.
—Jean Mayer.

According to the best available published figures, approximately one hundred eighty large multiphasic screening programs are operating in the United States at the present time.[1] There is considerable variation among them with regard to their purposes and, accordingly, the studied parameters. However, there is a glaring common deficit, namely, that diet is usually not considered.[1]

Without question diet and nutrition play an important role in the genesis of health and disease.[2] Additionally, abundant evidence exists to show that a significant segment of the American public is eating poorly.[3] In the light of these two well-recognized facts, *predictive medicine* differs from conventional medicine in that it incorporates dietary survey.

An attempt will be made in this chapter to demonstrate the utility of dietary analysis in the anticipation of diseases, many of which are *allegedly* nonnutritional syndromes.[4]

Diet and Clinical State

The literature is replete with evidence to show significant relationships between various classical disease syndromes and specific nutrients.[2] However, relatively little attention has been accorded the possible role of diet in the *early* stages of disease (chapter 4). For this reason, and only for illustrative purposes, one experiment will be cited here to underline a possible correlation between a *specific* nutrient and *general* symptoms and signs in a *presumably* healthy population.[4]

91

Two hundred twenty-one dentists and their wives participated in a survey in which each member completed a food frequency questionnaire. By computer analysis, a printout was provided showing the daily consumption of the major foodstuffs, the vitamins, the minerals, and comparisons with the Recommended Dietary Allowance provided by the Food and Nutrition Board of the National Research Council. For this example, only the daily vitamin C intake will be considered. Additionally, each participant completed the Cornell Medical Index Health Questionnaire. The number of positive responses, suggesting pathosis, was calculated and labeled CMI score.

Figure 9-1 shows age on the abscissa and the mean CMI scores on the ordinate. It is clear that, with age, the number of pathologic responses increases. Additionally, the subjects were divided into two groups based upon daily ascorbic acid intake. At every age group, the CMI scores are higher in the group consuming the lesser amount of vitamin C. Finally, it is noteworthy that the average intake of ascorbic acid, even in the poorer group, is well above the Recommended Dietary Allowance of 60 mg. per day.

This type of information, supported by other similar observations, suggests a correlation between diet and clinical findings characteristic of early disease stages.

Diet and Electrocardiography

It is well known that, with advancing age, there are electrocardiographic changes.[5] For example, with time, the height of the P wave in Lead I increases. Whether this is a physiologic aging phenomenon or a pathologic aging process that is characteristic of disease in the autumnal years is still argued. Suffice it to say however, that there is mounting evidence that the higher the P_1, the more pathologic is the picture.

Two hundred twenty-one presumably healthy subjects were studied in terms of daily thiamin intake and the height

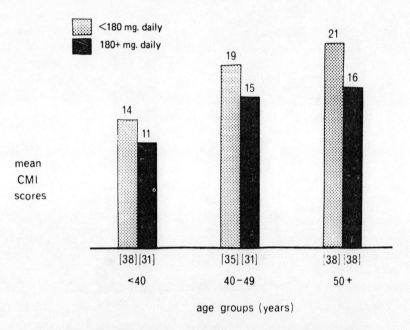

Figure 9-1. The relationship of age (on the abscissa) and number of clinical symptoms and signs (on the ordinate) in terms of daily vitamin C consumption. While symptoms and signs increase with time, the number at each age interval is higher in those consuming the lesser amounts of vitamin C (stippled columns).

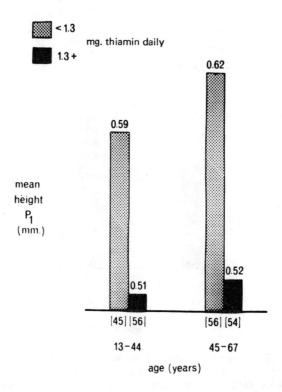

Figure 9-2. The relationship of age (on the x-axis) and height of P_1 (on the ordinate). The subjects consuming the lesser amounts of thiamin (stippled bars) show the tallest P_1 scores, particularly in the older age group.

of P_1.[4] Figure 9-2 pictorially portrays the results. Shown on the x-axis is age and on the y-axis the height of P_1. Generally speaking, the P_1 is higher in the older age group. However, the P wave is significantly higher in both age groups in those consuming the lower amounts of vitamin B_1 (stippled bars). These findings are in parallel with other reports showing, for example, the height and duration of P_1 with blood glucose.[6-7] Parenthetic mention should be made that a significant negative correlation (r = -0.385, P <0.05) was observed between P_1 height and blood glucose.

Thus, there is evidence that diet and various electrocardiographic parameters are closely related.

Diet and Biochemical State

Much is known about a number of nutrients and their relationship to various biochemical parameters. A classic example is carbohydrate intake and the glucose tolerance test. Actually, all nutrients are interrelated through their role in enzymes which regulate metabolism. Therefore, all nutrients are intimately related to the chemical constituents of the blood.

To underscore this point, and in an area not so clearly defined, figure 9-3 relates the parallelisms between daily vitamin E intake and nonfasting serum cholesterol levels. Two hundred twenty-eight males and 165 females, apparently healthy, were studied in terms of nonfasting serum cholesterol (on the vertical axis) and age (on the horizontal axis).[4] Additionally, both groups were subdivided into two subgroups based upon the daily vitamin E intake. The Food and Nutrition Board of the National Research Council recommends for the reference male a daily vitamin E intake of 30 I.U. Hence, shown in figure 9-3 are the males consuming less than 30 I.U. daily (stippled bars) and those consuming 30+ I.U. vitamin E (black columns).

The older males show higher cholesterol levels than the younger men. However, figure 9-3 also indicates that the

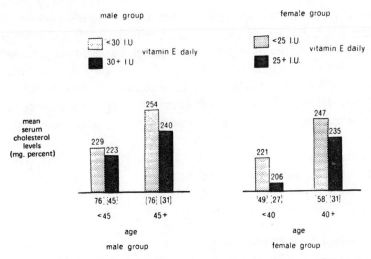

Figure 9-3. The relationship of age (on the horizontal axis) and nonfasting serum cholesterol (on the vertical axis). In both sexes, the subjects consuming the lesser amounts of vitamin E (stippled columns) show the relatively higher serum cholesterol values.

cholesterol scores are higher in those consuming the smaller amounts of vitamin E. According to the Food and Nutrition Board, the Recommended Dietary Allowances (RDA) for vitamin E are 25 I.U. for the female. Accordingly, figure 9-3 depicts the female groups based upon this delineation. It will be noted that the lower vitamin E intake parallels the higher serum cholesterol concentration. Thus, here is additional evidence that diet and the biochemical state are extensively interrelated.

Dietary Interrelationships

It is important to establish two additional points. First, nutrients are so well distributed in nature that a diet which is primarily composed of nutrient-rich calories (milk, cheese, meat, vegetables, fruit, nuts, whole-grain foods) supplies sufficient quantities of all essential nutrients (protein, vitamins, minerals). Thus, as the amount of food ingested goes up, so does the quantity of vitamins, minerals, and protein. In chapter 3 these nutrients were classified as resistance agents. Such factors decrease the likelihood of disease.

There is a high correlation between the amounts of nutrients ingested in a nourishing diet. Figure 9-4 demonstrates this for two essential nutrients in a study of 129 males and 82 females.[4] The daily vitamin B_1 and total protein consumption were determined by means of a food frequency questionnaire. Thiamin in milligrams is recorded on the abscissa and total protein intake in grams on the ordinate. The correlation coefficients of +0.769 for males and +0.713 for females attest to the statistically significant parallelisms in both sexes.

However, a diet composed of nutrient-rich calories may not be sufficient when there is a problem with the digestion,

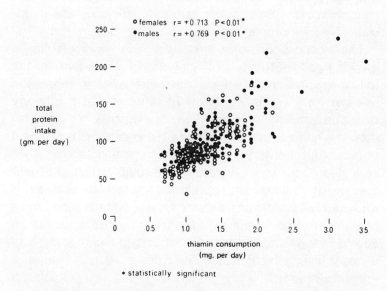

Figure 9-4. The relationship of daily thiamin (on the x-axis) and protein (on the y-axis) consumption. There are highly significant correlations in both sexes.

absorption, and utilization of nutrients. Also, there are many circumstances which bring about an increased requirement for one or more nutrients. Thus, flaws in assimilation and nutrient requirements would necessitate dietary nutrient supplementation. These are termed secondary deficiencies.

Second, subjects who consume large quantities of nutrient-poor calories receive lesser amounts of vitamins, minerals, and protein. For example, the person ingesting significant amounts of highly processed carbohydrate foods (including the "sweets") receives only a limited quantity of most essential nutrients from such foods. In addition, he has less appetite for more nourishing foods. In chapter 3 these nutrients were noted to be susceptibility factors. Such agents enhance the likelihood of disease.

A practical point to be considered from these examples and many other like observations is that it is rare, if not impossible, to find a *single* nutrient deficiency state generated by an improper diet.

The second point to be emphasized is that, metabolically speaking, all nutrients are interrelated as shown in the following citation: "Perhaps the most striking impression received from evaluation of the literature is that hardly any study undertaken with any pair of nutrients has failed to show a significant interrelation in terms of some nutritional or biochemical criterion. This is not surprising, though, since each step of the chain of reactions through which a nutrient goes as it follows an appropriate metabolic pathway is mediated by at least one enzyme system, and the functioning of every enzyme system calls for the combined action of an apoenzyme [made up for the most part of amino acids] and a coenzyme [which usually includes a vitamin and/or a mineral element]."[8]

Thus, single nutrient deficits from faulty assimilation or increased requirements do not occur. A shortage of one affects all the others through its role in metabolism.

Therefore, both dietary and nutritional imperfections

generate a multiple deficit rather than the shortage of a single essential nutrient.

Summary

One of the unique features of a predictive medicine program is its awareness of the role of diet in the anticipation of classical disease. This point is underlined with demonstrations of relationships between diet and clinical state, electrocardiographic parameters, and biochemical state. Additionally, the point is made that there are countless dietary interrelationships. As a result, it is not surprising that nutritional substances, metabolic reactions, and hormones are inseparably linked (figure 9-5).[9] What is particularly relevant is that certain nutrients may be viewed as *resistance* agents while other nutrients must be categorized as *susceptibility* factors, a subject which has been considered earlier (chapter 3).

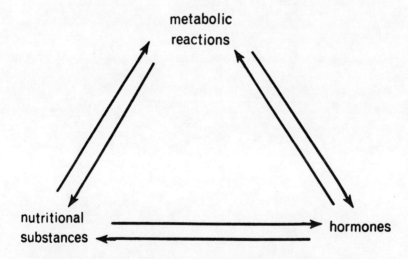

Figure 9-5. Schematic representation of the interplay of nutritional factors, hormones, and metabolism.

Predictive Medicine

References

1. Schoen, A. W. *Automated multiphasic health testing programs directory,* 1971-1972, second edition. Burbank, Bioscience Publications, Inc.

2. Cheraskin, E., Ringsdorf, W. M., Jr., and Clark, J. W. *Diet and disease.* 1968. Emmaus, Pennsylvania, Rodale Books.

3. United States Department of Agriculture. Agricultural Research Service. *Food consumption of households in the United States. Spring 1965. Household Food Consumption Survey.* Reports 1-5, 1968. Washington, D. C., United States Government Printing Office.

4. Cheraskin, E. and Ringsdorf, W. M., Jr. *Predictive medicine: IX. Diet.* J. Amer. Geriat. Soc. 19:11, 962-968, November 1971.

5. Lepeschkin, E. *Modern electrocardiography.* 1951. Baltimore, The Williams and Wilkens Company.

6. Cheraskin, E. and Ringsdorf, W. M., Jr. *Electrocardiography and carbohydrate metabolism: I. P-wave length (Lead I) in presumably healthy young men.* J. Med. Assn. St. Alabama 38:11, 1011-1014, May 1969.

7. Cheraskin, E. and Ringsdorf, W. M., Jr. *Electrocardiography and carbohydrate metabolism: II. P-wave height (Lead I) in presumably healthy young men.* Angiology 21:1, 18-23, January 1970.

8. Harte, R. A. and Chow, B. *Dietary interrelationships.* In Wohl, M. G. and Goodhart, R. S. *Modern nutrition in health and disease.* Third edition. 1964. Philadelphia, Lea and Febiger.

9. Dumm, M. E. and Ralli, E. P. *The hormonal control of metabolism.* In Wohl, M. G. and Goodhart, R. S. *Modern nutrition in health and disease.* Third edition. 1964. Philadelphia, Lea and Febiger.

Physical Activity

Those who think that they have not time for bodily exercise will sooner or later have to find time for illness.
        —Edward Stanley.

Without question medicine has attained a high degree of *technical* excellence for the management of many disease states. The wonders of plastic surgery and organ transplants are well-known. However, since little attention has been given to the *anticipation* and subsequent *prevention* of disease, particularly the chronic disorders (e.g., arthritis, cancer, heart disease), the therapeutic armamentarium is incomplete. Surely diet, a subject discussed in the previous chapter, is important. Another readily available and simply applied tool is physical activity. Surprisingly, except in isolated situations, exercise analysis and therapy are not a usual ingredient in multiple testing programs.[1] Thus, an appreciation of physical activity at the diagnostic and therapeutic levels adds to the uniqueness of a predictive medicine program.

Physical activity affects every aspect of body function—clinical, physiologic, and biochemical or metabolic. In this chapter examples will be given to demonstrate relationships between exercise and clinical symptoms and signs, electrocardiographic patterns, biochemical state, and parallelisms between exercise and variables such as coffee/tea, alcohol, tobacco consumption, and vitamin supplementation.[2]

Physical Activity and Clinical State

An increasing number of published reports deal with the utility of physical activity as it relates to mortality and to particular disease syndromes (e.g., ischemic heart disease,

10

hypertension, and diabetes mellitus).[3-5] For example, in a two year follow-up, men in every five-year age bracket between 45 and 84 years demonstrated an inverse relationship between exercise and mortality. A progressively lower death rate was observed as the degree of exercise increased.[3] Figure 10-1 illustrates this association in 50-54 year old men in four exercise groups.

However, there is only limited evidence to show the predictive value of exercise in terms of *early* clinical symptoms and signs.[6-7] Figure 10-2 demonstrates the relationship of age (on the abscissa) versus clinical symptoms and signs as judged from the Cornell Medical Index Health Questionnaire (on the ordinate) in terms of daily exercise.[2] Viewing figure 10-2 grossly, it is clear that the frequency of pathologic responses is significantly higher in both the younger and the older groups characterized by no daily exercise (black columns). Also, the difference in symptoms and signs in the older group is even more sharply defined in terms of daily physical activity. In other words, the progress of chronic disease appears to be considerably slowed in those who stay physically fit.

The relationship of physical activity and psychologic state has already been considered (chapter 3). It should be recalled that the number of psychologic findings in 208 dentists and their wives was 33 percent greater for the 126 persons who did not take daily exercise (figure 3-1).

Although many more examples could be cited, these simple observations are reasonable evidence of the predictive and preventive relationship of physical activity to the early clinical picture.

Physical Activity and Electrocardiography

It is generally agreed that, with advancing age, the height of the T wave in Lead I decreases.[8] To some, this is regarded as one measure of physiologic aging; to others this suggests pathosis. In support of the latter, there is reasonable evidence

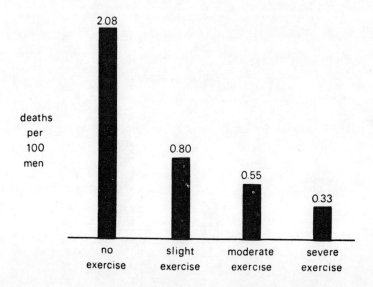

Hammond, E.C. <u>Some</u> <u>preliminary</u> <u>findings</u> <u>on</u>
<u>physical</u> <u>complaints</u> <u>from</u> a <u>prospective</u> <u>study</u>
<u>of</u> <u>1.064.004</u> <u>men</u> <u>and</u> <u>women</u>. Am. J. Public
Health 54: #1, 11-23, January 1964.

Figure 10-1. The relationship between physical activity and
mortality in 50-54-year-old men is an inverse one. The greater the
exercise the less was the mortality in a two-year follow-up.

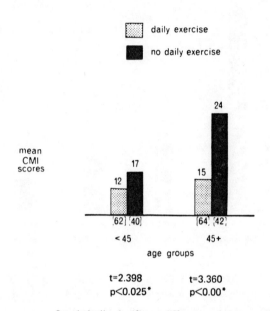

daily exercise

no daily exercise

mean
CMI
scores

24

17

12

15

[62] [40]   [64] [42]

< 45   45+

age groups

t=2.398   t=3.360
p<0.025*   p<0.00*

*statistically significant difference of the means

Figure 10-2. The relationship of age (on the abscissa) and clinical symptoms and signs as judged by CMI scores (on the ordinate) in terms of daily exercise. The groups, especially those in the older age category (45+ years), with no daily exercise show more clinical findings (black columns).

that, in certain cardiac disorders, the T wave is depressed.

The question at hand is whether there is any relationship between physical activity and the height of the T wave in presumably healthy subjects. Figure 10-3 pictorially portrays age on the x-axis and the mean height of T_1 on the y-axis in terms of daily exercise.[2] The evidence suggests that, particularly in the older age category (t = 2.052, P <0.05), there is a significant difference in the height of the T wave in those who report daily exercise versus those who do not. Specifi-

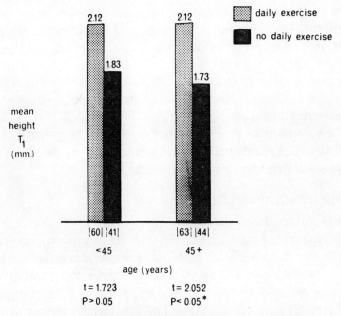

Figure 10-3. The relationship of age (on the x-axis) and mean height T_1 (on the ordinate) in terms of daily exercise. Those with daily exercise, and especially in the older age group (45+ years), show higher T_1 amplitude (stippled columns).

cally, the T wave is lower (more pathologic) in those without exercise (black column). For the physically fit in both age categories, the mean height of T_1 was the same.

This simple demonstration, supported by many others,[2] suggests that physical activity and various electrocardiographic parameters are related.

Physical Activity and Biochemical State

Increasing information indicates that blood glucose and serum cholesterol levels can be altered with physical activity. Although uric acid is in an area not usually considered, figure 10-4 shows the relationship between daily exercise and nonfasting serum uric acid levels.[2] The evidence suggests that, in a relatively older age sample, the serum uric acid level is significantly higher (t = 3.456, P <0.005) in subjects who do not carry on daily exercise. As noted for the CMI complaints (figure 10-2), there is little change with age in those who remain physically fit.

This demonstration, supported by others, suggests that a significant predictive-preventive relationship exists between physical activity and biochemical state.[2]

Physical Activity and Other Variables

Generally speaking, those who exercise are interested in the maintenance of health. Hence, it is interesting to observe other habits in subjects who perform daily exercise ·versus those who do not. Figure 10-5 is an analysis of the interplay of exercise and coffee/tea, alcohol, tobacco consumption, and vitamin supplementation.[2] The data suggest fewer people who carry out daily exercise drink coffee, tea, and alcohol. Most importantly, these individuals as a group consume much less tobacco. As a matter of fact, the number of nonexercising smokers is over threefold (23 to 7 percent) that observed in individuals who carry on daily physical activity. Finally, figure 10-5 shows that the frequency of vitamin supplementation is also greater in exercise groups.

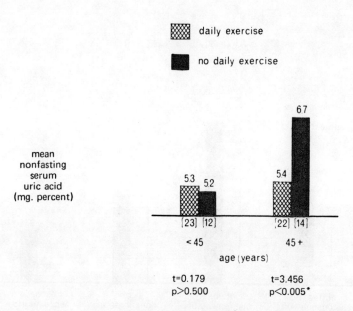

*statistically significant difference of the means

Figure 10-4. The relationship of age (on the horizontal axis) and serum uric acid scores (on the vertical axis). In the older group (45+ years), the group without daily exercise shows a statistically significantly higher mean nonfasting serum uric acid level (black column).

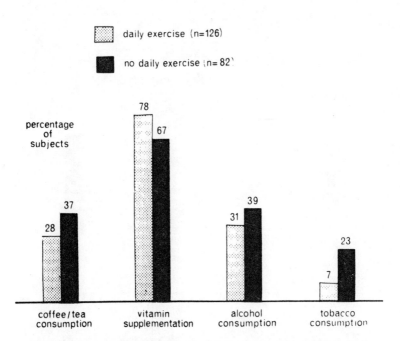

Figure 10-5. The interplay of exercise and other factors. It is noteworthy that subjects who exercise (stippled columns) tend to consume less coffee/tea, alcohol, tobacco and more frequently take vitamin supplements.

Summary

Earlier mention (chapter 3) has been made of factors which may be regarded as *susceptibility* versus *resistance* agents. Later, in chapter 9, it was established that certain dietary nutrients discourage the development of disease. Hence, they may be defined as *resistance* agents. Other dietary elements were noted to encourage disease. Accordingly, they may be viewed as *susceptibility* agents. The observations made in this report suggest that physical activity may be considered as a *resistance* factor. In other words, the addition of physical activity discourages disease; the absence of exercise invites disease.

The cardinal point to be made is that awareness of physical activity as it relates to the genesis of disease is a unique feature of a predictive medicine program.

References

1. Schoen, A. W. *Automated multiphasic health testing programs directory,* 1971-1972, second edition. Burbank, Bioscience Publications, Inc.

2. Cheraskin, E. and Ringsdorf, W. M., Jr. *Predictive medicine: X. Physical activity.* J. Amer. Geriat. Soc. 19:11, 969-973, November 1971.

3. Hammond, E. C. *Some preliminary findings on physical complaints from a prospective study of 1,064,004 men and women.* Amer. J. Pub. Health 54:1, 11-23, January 1964.

4. Cureton, T. K. *The physiological effects of exercise programs on adults.* 1969. Springfield, Charles C. Thomas.

5. Boyer, J. L. and Kasch, F. W. *Exercise therapy in hypertensive men.* J. A. M. A. 211:10, 1668-1671, 9 March 1970.

6. Brunner, D. and Jokl, E. *Physical activity and aging.* 1970. Baltimore, University Park Press.

7. Heinzelmann, F. and Bagley, R. W. *Response to physical activity programs and their effects on health behavior.* Pub. Health Rep. 85:10, 905-911, October 1970.

8. Lepeschkin, E. *Modern electrocardiography.* 1951. Baltimore, The Williams and Wilkens Company.

Prognostic Levels

In earlier chapters discussion has centered on clinical symptoms and signs, electrocardiographic parameters, biochemical state, enzymes, diet, physical activity, and genetics. The question now arises as to how these diverse parameters fit into a predictive scheme.

In conventional medicine the usual sequence of events includes a comparative analysis of a particular classical syndrome and its biochemical components. For example, in the traditional multiple testing program, considerable attention is directed to blood glucose levels as they relate to diabetes mellitus or serum cholesterol versus ischemic heart disease.

Predictive medicine, concerned as it is with the *anticipation* of disease, has given rise to a unique experimental model.[1] This is another feature which sets predictive medicine apart from conventional medicine.

Anatomy of Man in a Predictive Medicine System

Man may be viewed as a multilamellated sphere.[2-4] Any way one turns a ball, it looks the same. In a sense, however one diagnostically inspects man from the outside, the predictability is the same. True, viewed on one side, there may be a limp characteristic of a cerebrovascular accident; examined from a different angle, there are pimples. But these and all other peripheral stigmata have a common denominator; they

110

signify an index of the syndrome of sickness (figure 11-1).

Additionally, as progressively deeper layers of the lamellated sphere are examined, one eventually approaches the core. In man also, diagnostic layers may be stripped away until the central problems are brought into focus (figure 11-1).

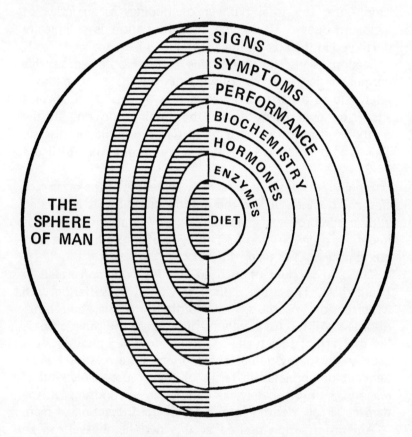

Figure 11-1. Man may be likened to a lamellated sphere. The peripheries of both are easily inspected. Layers can be removed which progressively expose the core problems.

Signs. The outer, most peripheral, ring is readily inspected in both a sphere and in man. At this level, one can make three observations.

First (in incipient stages), it is possible to establish simply the numbers and kinds of signs without any regard to how or why they fit into systems or sites. In other words, one can simply use the total number of findings as an index of incipient disease. This type of information is graphically portrayed in the box on the left (figure 11-2).

Second, signs and symptoms can be obtained at this peripheral level which provide an estimate of pathosis referrable to a particular system (e.g., gastrointestinal) or a site (e.g., eye) even though the findings do not fit the textbook description of a particular syndrome or disease. This type of information is shown in the center box of figure 11-2.

Finally, it is possible to identify evidences of the ravages of *classical* disease such as the pathognomonic gait associated with a cerebrovascular accident, a skin eruption typical of impetigo, a carious tooth. This type of information fits the box on the right in figure 11-2.

The end product of such an analysis is demonstrated in figure 11-3. Thus, the patient is viewed as suffering with hypertension, psoriasis, periodontitis, myopia, and other disorders. All too frequently many of these and other chronic ills that afflict society have a poorly defined etiology. It is usually the opinion that these diseases are relatively independent or unrelated in terms of their causes. This kind of *diagnosis,* unfortunately, is simply an accounting of the damage largely derived from a peripheral inspection of man.

Any information desired at this peripheral level can be readily derived by physical examination and through history taking.

Symptoms. If one strips off the outer layer (figure 11-1), into focus comes the zone of symptoms. Alterations of taste, smell, hearing, sight, and touch may be reported as symp-

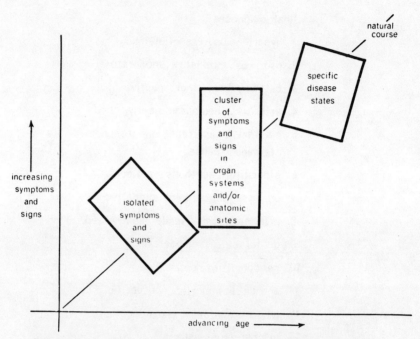

Figure 11-2. The periphery of man provides three sets of information: first, the early and seemingly unrelated findings (box on the left), symptoms and signs in systems and sites (box in the middle), and the presence of obvious classical diseases (box on the right).

Doe   Jane   47   W F

final diagnoses

1. hypertension, essential, mild

2. psoriasis, exfoliative, moderate

3. osteomyelitis, femur, inactive

4. arthritis, rheumatoid, early

5. epistaxis, recurrent, due to unde-
    termined cause

6. stomatitis, aphthous, periodic

7. emphysema, chronic, idiopathic

8. arteriosclerosis, senile, generalized

9. dental caries, moderate

10. periodontitis, nonspecific

11. anemia, normocytic, nonspecific

12. gastritis, chronic, idiopathic

13. myopia, progressive

14. psychoneurosis, mild

Figure 11-3. A typical diagnostic workup showing an array of problems having as a common denominator unknown etiology.

toms. However, where the outer layer ends and the next most peripheral one begins can be quite arbitrary. Also, the designation of whether a finding is a symptom or a sign is very flexible. For example, bleeding when observed by a doctor is classified as a sign but would be regarded as a symptom when reported by the patient.

Symptoms are not as readily discernable as signs and can only be derived through interrogation by means of a classical interview or questionnaire (e.g., the reporting of headaches, pain, or burning sensations in the mouth). Analysis of symptoms is regarded by some investigators as an important tool in the prediction of illness. The important point to be recognized, for predictive purposes, is that symptoms generally *precede* signs of disease. Hence, evidence obtained in this zone may be regarded as *prognostic*.

Performance. Stripping off the second layer unearths the world of performance (figure 11-1). Impairment in performance generally heralds the appearance of symptoms and signs. The malfunction begins in cells but eventually encompasses a tissue, organ, or system. Such information can be elicited from questionnaires, physical performance, organ, and system performance evaluations. Physical activity is frequently used in the evaluation of organ and system activity (e.g., the treadmill in the assessment of the cardiovascular system). The important point to underline is that a disturbance in performance precedes symptoms and signs of disease. Hence, this zone can be used very effectively in a predictive medicine program.

Biochemical state. Removing the performance layer brings into view the biochemical pattern. This is a very complex, yet productive, area, and the number of items that could be subjected to analysis is endless. Blood chemical determinations such as glucose or cholesterol are good examples. Biochemical tests on saliva, urine, and breath also provide significant diagnostic data.

This lamella is predictive of the three peripheral zones

115

since biochemical imbalance antedates disturbances in performance and the advent of symptoms and signs. Thus, chemical diabetes mellitus, characterized by disturbances in blood glucose, precedes the clinical diabetic syndrome by months and even years (chapter 4).

Hormonal balance. Dissecting off the biochemical layer brings into view the deeper hormonal area. It is here that measures of endocrine state (e.g., protein-bound iodine) are disclosed. Aberrations in hormonal state may precede changes in biochemical homeostasis. For example, the hypothyroid patient frequently demonstrates hypercholesterolemia, and hyperadrenal cortical activity is reflected by changes in blood glucose or electrolytes. Hence, hormonal imbalances become predictive of the more peripheral layers because they contribute to metabolic disturbances.

Enzymes. At the near center of the core is the enzyme pattern. Many of the 2,000 known enzymes can be measured. For example, serum glutamic oxalacetic transaminase (SGOT) is now frequently utilized as a predictive tool of impending cardiovascular disease. Since metabolism is made possible because of enzymes, enzymatic imbalance can be predictive of changes in the peripheral layers.

The core problems. Finally, one reaches the core which in figure 11-1 is illustrated by diet. Since dietary nutrients are the building blocks from which enzymes and hormones are made, it is apparent that all the peripheral layers reveal the effects of dietary imbalances, inadequacies, or excesses. As has been pointed out earlier, physical fitness can also be regarded as a core problem. Surely, genetics must always be considered. Finally, other core variables receiving increasing attention are pollutants, preservatives in foods, et cetera.

When there are no core problems, and especially when an optimal diet exists, all peripheral layers are in order. Thus, in the healthy man, all levels are in balance (figure 11-4).

On the other hand, when there is a core problem, such as a poor diet, there are reverberations throughout all diagnostic levels. This begins in the more central area of enzyme balance and proceeds in order to the peripheral signs and symptoms (figure 11-5).

A Practical Application

Each of the diagnostic levels (signs, symptoms, performance, biochemistry, hormones, enzymes, and diet) is interrelated with every other level. Thus, the predictive value is greatly enhanced. For example, number of hours of sleep versus mortality has been studied[6] (chapter 5). It was observed that both too little and too much sleep (symptoms) affect the core variable, physical fitness, by increasing mortality (figure 5-3). Another such observation is reported here[1] which links physical fitness as a core problem with the more peripheral estimates of signs and symptoms (sick call) as shown in figure 11-1.

The Officers Candidate School (OCS) at Fort Benning, Georgia, consists of an intensive twenty-four-week training program. At the start of the course each student is graded with a variety of mental and physical tests. One of the measuring procedures is the time required to run one mile. During the subsequent twenty-four-week training period, a record is kept of military and medical parameters indicating the number of times each student reports for sick call. Figure 11-6 pictorially portrays the relationship of the time required to run one mile (on the x-axis) and the frequency of sick call (on the y-axis) in 392 soldiers deemed healthy enough to be trained for officer status. Those individuals who run the mile fastest *at the start of the program* are the very same persons who *subsequently* report least for sick call. Conversely, those with the *longest* initial scores for the mile run are characterized by the *highest* sick call frequency. Thus, those with the best performance, as judged by the mile run, subsequently demonstrate the least number of peripheral problems (figure 11-4). Those with the poorest performance record display the most symptoms and signs (figure 11-5).

117

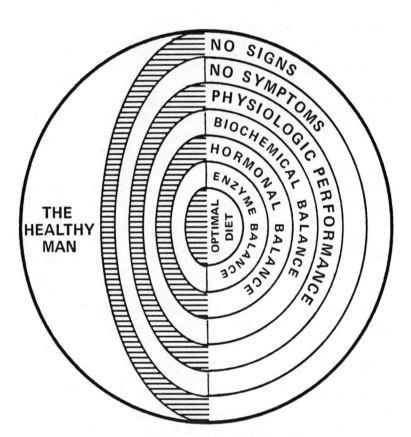

Figure 11-4. In healthy man all levels are in balance.

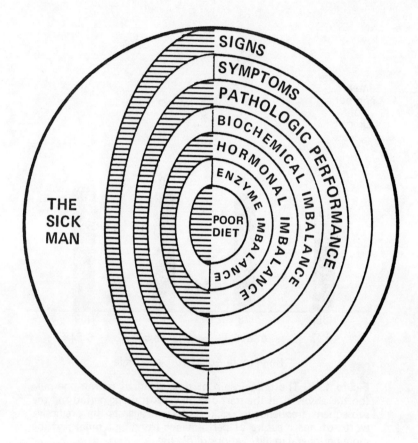

Figure 11-5. Following a core problem (diet, exercise, et cetera), there are eventual disturbances in order at the enzyme level, hormones, biochemical state, performance, and finally symptoms and signs.

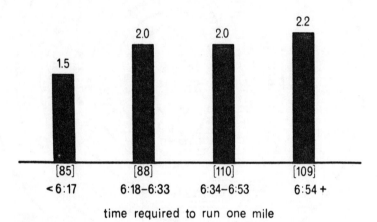

Figure 11-6. The relationship of time required to run one mile (on the abscissa) at the start of a 24-week training period and the subsequent frequency of sick call. This suggests the predictive worth of one measure of performance (running a mile) and the more peripheral manifestations of disease.

These experimental findings are consistent with the report of a negative association between degree of exercise and death in men 45 to 85+ years of age.[6] In other words, as the degree of exercise increased from none to slight, moderate, and heavy, deaths decreased progressively. Between no exercise and heavy exercise the differences ranged from fivefold to tenfold.

Summary

An analysis of the periphery of man (symptoms and signs) is useful in that it provides a measure of the extent of disease. However, in itself, it has little utility in a predictive medicine program. The present methods of correlation of biochemical state and symptoms and signs, characteristic of existing multiple testing programs, are helpful in the diagnosis of classical disease. However, its predictive potential is limited. A predictive medicine program, to fulfill its true purpose, must view the total sphere and identify the relative prognosticative potential of the different interrelated layers.

References

1. Cheraskin, E. and Ringsdorf, W. M., Jr. *Predictive medicine: XI. Prognostic levels.* J. Amer. Geriat. Soc. 19:12, 1000-1005, December 1971.
2. Cheraskin, E. and Ringsdorf, W. M., Jr. *The health of the dentist and his wife: a predictive health program.* J. South. California Dent. Assn. 37:7, 271-276, July 1969.
3. Cheraskin, E. and Ringsdorf, W. M., Jr. *The health of the dentist and his wife: present findings in a predictive health program.* J. South. California Dent. Assn. 37:9, 413-421, September 1969.
4. Cheraskin, E. *Concepts in predictive medicine.* Lab News 11:2, 23-26, August 1970.
5. Katcher, A. H. Personal communication. Philadelphia, University of Pennsylvania, School of Dental Medicine.
6. Hammond, E. C. *Some preliminary findings on physical complaints from a prospective study of 1,064,004 men and women.* Amer. J. Pub. Health 54:1, 11-23, January 1964.

Oral Cavity

The condition and functioning of the teeth and periodontium are not of self-contained importance; their state of health implicates all the rest of the body.
—Sperber.

Earlier mention was made that existing multiple testing programs assign little or no value to diet (chapter 10) and physical activity (chapter 11) in the genesis of *early* disease. A third area which is usually slighted is the oral cavity.[1] This is another unique feature of a predictive medicine program, for it recognizes that the mouth is a vital, integral part of the total organism.[2]

Mortality and the Teeth

A number of interesting observations suggest that the body dies in toto. For example, there is evidence that the oral cavity ages and "dies" in parallel with the rest of the organism. Thus, much valuable predictive data can be derived from a study of the oral tissues.

In a recent study[3] life expectancy was found to be closely related to the number of permanent teeth in 2,116 presumably healthy subjects. Figure 12-1 shows that the mean number of teeth (continuous line) rises to 27 at the mean age of 24 and progressively declines to an average of five at age 64. An extrapolation backward (interrupted line) to zero teeth crosses the horizontal axis at five years of age. Interestingly enough, this is consistent with the initial eruption time of the permanent teeth. If one may assume that total edentulousness represents oral death and that oral and bodily death should be related, then projecting the pattern (interrupted line) with advancing age shows that the point (on the abscissa) at which the average subject is expected to be *without all teeth* is approximately 70-71

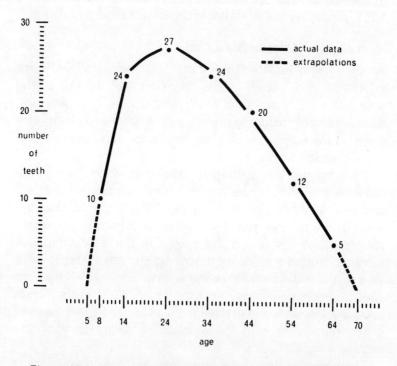

Figure 12-1. The relationship of age (on the abscissa) and mean number of permanent teeth (on the ordinate) as shown by the continuous line. The extrapolation (interrupted line) back indicates that no permanent teeth are present at approximately age five. This is consistent with well-known clinical observations. The extrapolation (interrupted line) forward anticipates no teeth in all subjects at age 70.5 years. This is consistent with the average life expectancy in the United States.

years. It is particularly noteworthy that the highest estimated expectation of life at birth ever recorded in the United States—70.5 years for the total population—was attained in 1967, according to the National Center for Health Statistics.[4]

Mortality and Alveolar Bone Loss

While it must be admitted that the above parallelisms are interesting and interrelate the dentition with the rest of the organism, it is clear that tooth loss occurs for many and diverse reasons including unnecessary extractions. Thus, in a given individual there may be no association between oral and systemic collapse.

To validate the data just described and obviate the objections which may be raised, an analysis was made of age and alveolar bone height.[2] Figure 12-2 depicts the relationship of mean age (on the x-axis) and mean percentage alveolar bone height (on the y-axis) in the same sample of subjects utilized for the tooth loss experiment.[3] The point at which it is anticipated that the average subject will have *no* tooth supporting osseous tissues is about 70-71 years. This is precisely the same age derived from a study of tooth loss and quite in keeping with the average life expectancy of the average American.

The common denominator in both of these observations is that the mouth reflects the health status of the total organism and should be incorporated in any total health evaluation system.

Morbidity and the Oral Cavity

While the relationships just shown are interesting, they are purely philosophic *mortality* projections. The question arises as to whether comparable *morbidity* parallelisms prevail. The categoric answer is that there are countless interrelationships between oral health and that of the total organism.

A simple tooth count is not only interrelated with longevity but is prognostic of morbidity. Barach[5] analyzed

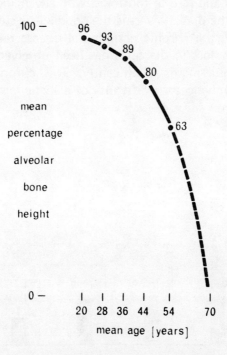

Figure 12-2. The relationship of age (on the horizontal axis) and mean percentage alveolar bone height (on the vertical axis) as observed (continuous line). The extrapolation (interrupted line) suggests that, at age 70.5 years, no alveolar bone height is expected in the population. This is consistent with the average life expectancy in the United States.

the mean number of teeth in various age groups in 200 diabetic subjects and 12,000 individuals who, in his opinion, could be regarded as nondiabetic. Figure 12-3 shows quite clearly that the rate of tooth loss with advancing age is much greater in the diabetic versus the nondiabetic subject. On the other hand, the chronic periodontal disease responsible for most tooth loss in diabetics has been observed to increase insulin requirements significantly. This chronic infection, therefore, enhances the difficulty of diabetic regulation.[6]

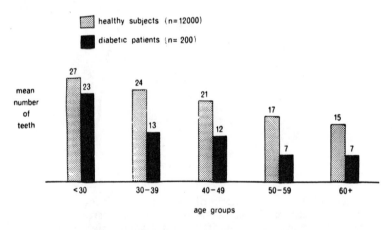

Barach, J. H. Diabetes and its treatment. 1949. New York, Oxford University Press. p. 90.

Figure 12-3. The relationship of age and tooth loss in 200 diabetic subjects (black columns) and 12,000 nondiabetic individuals (stippled columns). The rate of tooth loss with age is much greater in patients with diabetes mellitus.

Even in nondiabetic subjects, there are significant relationships between blood glucose and various oral parameters. In one such study,[7] the relationship of age and alveolar bone loss in terms of fasting blood glucose was investigated in 119 subjects (figure 12-4). Alveolar bone loss was graded on radiographs by a seven-point scale from 0 (no loss) to 6 (total loss). Within the limits of this experiment, the relationship between alveolar bone loss and age is greatest in the relatively hypoglycemic individuals (r = +0.501, P <0.01). Next in order, alveolar bone loss and age correlate most significantly in the relatively hyperglycemic (r = +0.429, P <0.01). Finally, the lowest correlation appears in the relatively normoglycemic (r = +0.359, P <0.05). This, it should be recalled, underlines the parabolic concept earlier described (chapter 5).

The point has been made in the last two examples that there appear to be relationships between oral parameters and general health as determined by biochemical tests. Additional evidence of oral and general health correlations occur at the clinical level.

Figure 12-5 describes a study of 1,288 presumably healthy individuals[8] who completed the Cornell Medical Index Health Questionnaire (CMI). The reliability and validity of data so derived has been recognized.[9-10] Parenthetic mention should be made that the questionnaire includes only three dental questions:

1. Have you lost more than half your teeth?
2. Are you troubled by bleeding gums?
3. Have you often had severe toothaches?

An analysis was made of the frequency of positive dental complaints versus general health findings. The frequency of dental findings in those individuals characterized by more than fifty positive responses on the Cornell Medical Index Health Questionnaire is pictured on the top line of figure 12-5. The pattern is of interest for two reasons. The group characterized by the greatest frequency of general complaints

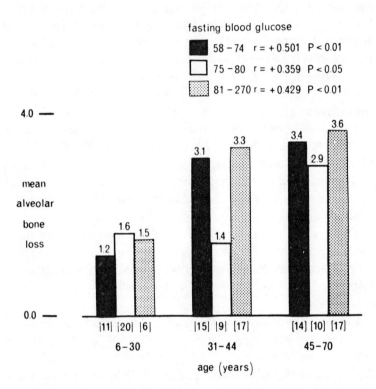

Figure 12-4. The relationship of age (x-axis) and alveolar bone loss (y-axis) in terms of fasting blood glucose. The highest correlation (r = +0.501, P <0.01) is between age and alveolar bone loss (black columns) in the relative hypoglycemic (58-74 mg. percent) group. The next highest relationship (r = +0.429, P <0.01) between age and alveolar bone loss (stippled columns) is found in the relative hyperglycemic group (81-270 mg. percent). The lowest correlation (r = +0.359, P <0.05) in noted (white columns) in the relative normoglycemic category (75-80 mg. percent).

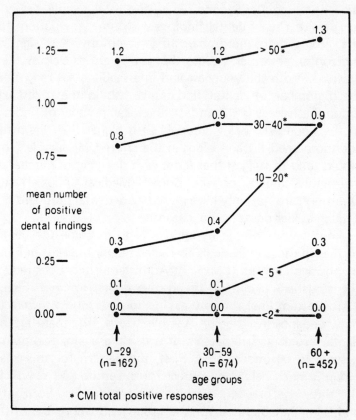

Figure 12-5. The relationship of age (on the horizontal axis) to mean number of positive dental findings (on the vertical axis) in terms of reported general symptoms and signs as derived from the Cornell Medical Index Health Questionnaire in 1288 presumably healthy individuals. In the subjects with the least number of general findings (<2) there are no dental findings in any of the age groups (bottom line). In the group with the greatest number of general symptoms and signs (>50), there are the most dental findings in all age groups (top line). The intermediate groups in terms of general findings occupy intermediate positions in terms of dental symptoms and signs.

shows dental findings distinctly above the average trend for the entire sample. Second, while the total sample shows a progressive rise of dental findings with time, the pattern for the group with more than fifty symptoms and signs is horizontal. In other words, the young are as sick as their elders. In both the youngest and intermediate age ranges the mean number of dental findings is 1.2; in the oldest age group the average is 1.3. In fact, the mean number of findings in the youngest "sick" group (1.2) is higher than the mean for those aged 60 and older in the entire CMI sample. This would tend to suggest that those with the greatest number of affirmative replies on the Cornell Medical Index Health Questionnaire not only have more severe dental problems but a much earlier onset of oral pathosis.

Another test of the hypothesis is to examine the dental picture in those individuals characterized by the least number of positive answers (CMI <2). Admittedly, this does reduce the statistical likelihood of positive dental findings. Figure 12-5 (bottom line) shows that, in those persons with zero or only one positive finding (sample size = 14), there are no dental problems irrespective of age. Here again, two points deserve to be underscored. First, the pattern for this small group is much below the average for the entire CMI sample in the three age brackets. Second, this trend is also horizontal and, like that pictured for the group with more than fifty positive answers, does not change with age.

These are the two extremes, the obviously ill and the optimally healthy. The point now to be established is the pattern for the person who is minimally or marginally sick. Shown in figure 12-5 is the trend for three such intermediate groups.

It will be noted that the least sick of these groups (<5 positive replies) demonstrates a dental finding pattern (increasing severity with age) analogous but slightly more severe than that of the group with <2 positive CMI responses. On the other hand, the somewhat sicker intermediate group

(30-40 positive replies) demonstrates the horizontal dental finding pattern, though less severe, of the sickest group.

Finally, if dental findings may be regarded as a measure of biologic age, the positive responses for the three chronologic age groups take on added significance. Specifically, it will be noted that within each CMI group (as measured by total positive CMI responses) those aged 60 and over are, biologically speaking, approximately as young as or younger than those in the zero to 29-year-age range of the next "sickest" group. For example, the mean number of positive dental findings for those 60+ with a CMI <5 is identical to that of the youngest age range with a CMI of 10-20. Comparable relationships can be made between the other groups.

The Oral Cavity in an Ecosystem

Mention was made earlier (chapter 3) that whether one remains healthy or becomes ill is a function of the environment *and* host state. Accordingly, it is relevant to examine the relationship of the oral cavity to general health in this ecosystem.

Figure 12-6 describes the mean gingival disease scores on the ordinate in terms of number of general symptoms and signs and frequency of toothbrushing on the abscissa.[11] It will be observed that the highest mean gingival score (0.69), and therefore the most pathologic, appears in the group characterized by the greater number of CMI responses (7+) and the lesser amount of toothbrushing (1-2 times per day). Conversely, the lowest mean gingival score (0.48), and therefore the most physiologic pattern, is noted in the group characterized by the lesser number of general symptoms and signs (0.6) and the greater toothbrushing (3+ daily). Finally, the two intermediate groups in terms of mean gingival scores are the same (0.56) and represent those with the fewer general complaints and lesser toothbrushing and the greater number of general findings and greater toothbrushing. This simple experiment underlines the relationship between the

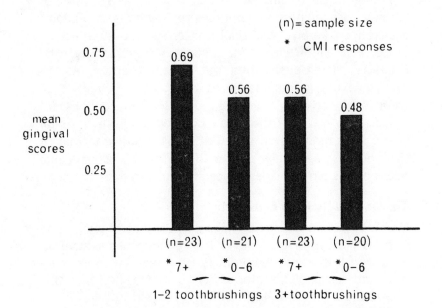

Figure 12-6. The relationship of gingival state (on the ordinate) and general findings and toothbrushing frequency (on the abscissa). The highest, and therefore poorest mean gingival score is noted in the group with the greater number of general symptoms and signs (7+) and in those with the lesser toothbrushing (1-2 times per day). The lowest, and consequently best mean gingival score is observed in the group with the fewer number of general findings (0-6) and with the greater toothbrushing frequency (3+ times per day). The intermediate groups in terms of gingival state are the same characterized by fewer brushings and better general health and greater number of brushings and poorer general health.

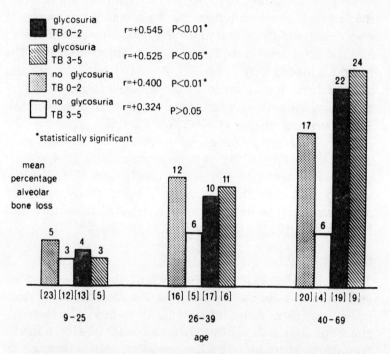

Figure 12-7. Relationship of age (on the x-axis) and alveolar bone loss (on the y-axis) in terms of daily toothbrushing frequency and glycosuria. The highest correlation (r = +0.545, P <0.01) occurs in those brushing relatively little (0-2 times per day) and with glycosuria (black columns). The lowest correlation (r = +0.324, P >0.05) is noted in the group with greater toothbrushing (3-5 times per day) and no glycosuria (white columns).

environment, in this case as judged by toothbrushing, and host state as evaluated by CMI responses in terms of oral health (gingival state).

To complete the story, figure 12-7 pictures the relationship of host state (as judged by the presence or absence of glycosuria) and daily toothbrushing frequency as it relates to alveolar bone loss in 149 apparently healthy subjects.[7] The highest correlation (r = +0.545, P <0.01) between age and alveolar bone loss is noted in the subjects characterized by glycosuria and relatively little toothbrushing (black columns). The lowest correlation (r = +0.324, P >0.05) appears in the group with no glycosuria and more toothbrushing (white columns). The other two combinations occupy intermediate positions in terms of correlation coefficients. Thus, pathologic aging as exemplified by alveolar bone loss proceeds at a much slower rate in those with relatively satisfactory oral hygiene and efficient carbohydrate metabolism.

Summary

The oral cavity is an integral part of the total organism. Hundreds of publications attest to the fact that the mouth influences general health and vice versa.[12-15] Notwithstanding, it is noteworthy that rarely are the oral tissues considered in multiple testing programs. Hence, because of the evidence shown in this report, predictive medicine is unique in that it utilizes the oral cavity as one prognostic tool.

References

1. Schoen, A. W. *Automated multiphasic health testing programs directory,* 1971-1972, second edition. Burbank, Bioscience Publications, Inc.

2. Cheraskin, E. and Ringsdorf, W. M., Jr. *Predictive medicine: XII. Oral cavity.* J. Amer. Geriat. Soc. 20:2, 88-92, February 1972.

3. Cheraskin, E. and Ringsdorf, W. M., Jr. *Aging by the teeth.* Lancet 1:7594, 580, 15 March 1969.

4. *Medical Scene: Life expectancy up.* Mod. Med. 36:18, 42, 26 August 1968.

5. Barach, J. H. *Diabetes and its treatment.* 1949. New York, Oxford University Press. p. 90.

6. Williams, R. C., Jr. and Mahan, C. J. *Periodontal disease and diabetes in young adults.* J. A. M. A. 172:8, 776-778, 20 February 1960.

7. Cheraskin, E. and Ringsdorf, W. M., Jr. *Ecology of alveolar bone loss.* Oral Surg., Oral Med., Oral Path. 30:3, 333-350, September 1970.

8. Cheraskin, E., Ringsdorf, W. M., Jr., Setyaadmadja, A. T. S. H., and Barrett, R. A. *Predictive dentistry: the Cornell Medical Index Health Questionnaire (general response) and dental findings.* New York J. Dent. 37:3, 104-107, March 1967.

9. Meltzer, J. W. and Hochstim, J. R. *Reliability and validity of survey data on physical health.* Pub. Health Rep. 85:12, 1075-1086, December 1970.

10. Alexiou, N. G., Wiener, G., Silverman, M., and Milton, T. *Validity studies of a self-administered health questionnaire for secondary school students.* Amer. J. Pub. Health 59:8, 1400-1412, August 1969.

11. Cheraskin, E. and Ringsdorf, W. M., Jr. *The dental hygienist in health evaluation.* J. Amer. Dent. Hygien. Assn. 42:3, 151-154, Third Quarter 1968.

12. Sandler, H. C. and Stahl, S. S. *The influence of generalized diseases on clinical manifestations of periodontal disease.* J. A. D. A. 49:6, 656-667, December 1954.

13. Muhler, J. C. *The oral tissues: the barometer of the body.* J. A. D. A. 61:3, 301-307, September 1960.

14. Sperber, G. H. *Interrelationship of oral and general health.* J. Canad. Dent. Assn. 31:11, 725-731, November 1965.

15. United States Department of Health, Education, and Welfare, Public Health Service. *Selected examination findings related to periodontal disease among adults, United States 1960-1962.* National Center for Health Statistics, Series 11:33. Washington, U. S. Government Printing Office.

Tolerance Testing

Testing under load or stress conditions may be likened to getting a young doctor drunk the morning he takes his state board examinations. The results may be revealing. However, the purpose of the state board is to establish how he will fare under the usual practice conditions, and it is hoped that he will usually not be intoxicated.   —Cheraskin.

There is increasing interest in the utility of testing under load or stress conditions for diagnostic and prognostic purposes. This is underscored by the various exercise procedures prior to electrocardiography and by the stressing techniques (preparatory diet, glucose loading, glucose-steroid load) employed for assessment of glucose tolerance.[1] There is no question but that these pretest conditions have yielded much valuable diagnostic information.

However, in a predictive medicine program designed to *anticipate* rather than *identify* disease, tolerance testing should be viewed critically. First, for many people, the test circumstances are abnormal. What one wishes to learn in a predictive medicine system is how the subject is coping with his everyday problems. Second, tolerance testing simply exaggerates the metabolic flaw and makes classical diagnosis easier or more convincing. Third, the very same information derived under tolerance conditions can be obtained without loading if one is willing to accept the fact that physiologic and normal values are not the same and that small changes in a particular parameter are significant. These concepts have been dealt with in chapters 2 through 6.

An attempt will be made in this chapter to show the relative utility of tolerance and nontolerance tests for

13

136

predictive purposes employing blood glucose as the experimental model.[2]

Tolerance Tests

The most popular load technique performed in conventional medicine today is the glucose tolerance test. Figure 13-1 is an analysis of this procedure in 120 presumably healthy subjects.[3] Fasting blood glucose groups have been created in

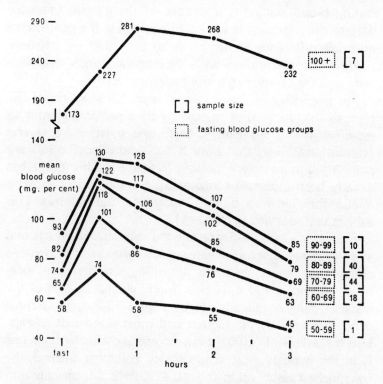

Figure 13-1. The classical glucose tolerance test in 120 presumably healthy subjects. The pre-load (fasting) scores are predictive of the post-load (1/2, 1, 2, and 3 hours) values.

10 mg. percent increments (in the boxes at the right). For example, there is one subject in the 50-59 mg. percent group with a fasting blood glucose of 58 mg. percent (sample size is shown in brackets on the right). There are 18 subjects in the 60-69 mg. percent group with a mean fasting blood glucose of 65 mg. percent. Figure 13-1 graphically shows that the subsequent mean blood glucose levels (1/2, 1, 2, and 3 hours) *after* glucose loading are directly related to the *fasting* concentration. Specifically, the higher the fasting score, the higher are the values following loading with glucose. Hence, fasting blood glucose is predictive of the glucose tolerance pattern provided one is willing to appreciate the significance of small differences (chapters 4 to 6). Other reports have confirmed these findings with the classical glucose tolerance test[4] and the cortisone glucose tolerance test.[2]

For predictive purposes certain *temporal* segments of the glucose tolerance curve appear to be superior. In order to establish which segment is best, one must make several assumptions. First, that both hyper- and hypoglycemia are pathologic; normoglycemia is physiologic. This point has already been discussed (chapter 5). Second, that there is a relationship between blood glucose and oral pathosis. This subject was reviewed in chapter 12.

Figures 13-2 to 13-6 portray the relationship of age and alveolar bone loss, as measured by one of the available clinical techniques, in terms of fasting, one-half-hour, one-hour, two-hour, and three-hour blood glucose as part of the classical glucose tolerance test.[2] Figure 13-2 suggests three conclusions. First, the highest and most significant correlation (r = +0.501, P <0.01) between age and alveolar bone loss is in the hypoglycemic group (black columns). Second, the next highest relationship (r = +0.429, P <0.01) prevails with the hyperglycemic group (stippled columns). Finally, there is even a significant correlation (r = +0.359, P <0.05) between age and alveolar bone loss in the normoglycemic category (white columns). In short, it appears that fasting blood

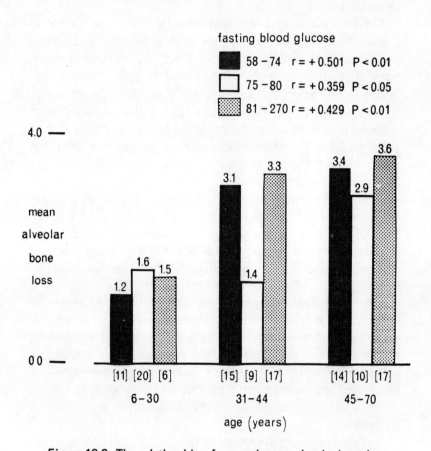

Figure 13-2. The relationship of age and mean alveolar bone loss in terms of fasting blood glucose. Statistically significant correlations exist in all three groups (hyper-, normo-, and hypoglycemia) with the highest correlation in the hypoglycemic and the lowest in the normoglycemic group.

glucose can serve in a predictive system but with a low sensitivity level.

Figure 13-3 relates age and alveolar bone loss to blood glucose recorded thirty minutes after a glucose load. Three points warrant special attention. First, the pattern is essentially that observed with fasting blood glucose (figure 13-2). Second, the hyper- and hypoglycemic correlations are higher than observed in the fasting state. Third, the relationship of normoglycemia to age and alveolar bone loss is not significant ($r = +0.243$, $P > 0.05$). Hence, it would appear that the thirty-minute blood glucose is more predictive than the fasting determination.

Figure 13-4 analyzes the relationship of age and alveolar bone loss to the blood glucose one hour after glucose loading. The highest and most significant correlation is found in the normoglycemic group ($r = +0.483$, $P < 0.01$). Therefore, the one-hour post-load blood glucose has no prognosticative value within the limits of these observations.

Figure 13-5 relates age and alveolar bone loss to two-hour (post-loading) blood glucose. There are significant parallelisms with both hyper- and hypoglycemia and none with normoglycemia giving this test a high degree of predictive value. Finally, the three-hour post-load picture shows a significant correlation with all three glucose groups (figure 13-6). Thus, the three-hour level is disqualified for predictive purposes.

Detailed comparative study of figures 13-2 to 13-6 suggests that the most predictive temporal point in the glucose tolerance test appears to be *two hours* after glucose loading (figure 13-5). Four reasons are noteworthy. First, the rate of alveolar bone loss with age is not statistically significant for the normoglycemic group ($r = +0.245$, $P > 0.05$). Second, the hypoglycemic correlation ($r = +0.531$, $P < 0.01$) is exceeded only by the one-half and three-hour groups. Third, the hyperglycemic correlation is higher than at any other temporal point ($r = +0.500$, $P < 0.01$). Finally, it is

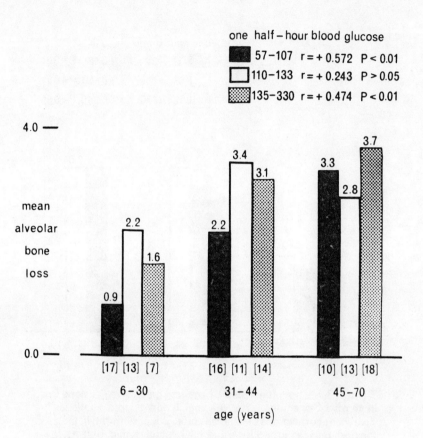

Figure 13-3. The relationship of age and mean alveolar bone loss in terms of thirty-minute (after loading) blood glucose. Statistically significant correlations exist only in the hypo- and hyperglycemic groups with the highest correlation in the group with relatively low blood glucose.

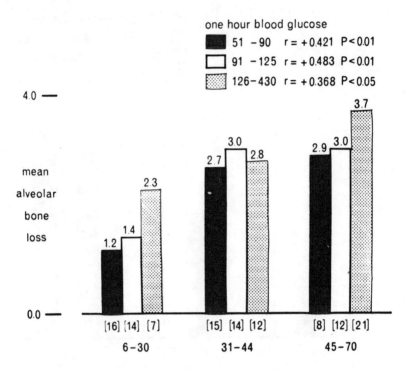

Figure 13-4. The relationship of age and mean alveolar bone loss in terms of one-hour (after loading) blood glucose. Statistically significant correlations exist in all three groups with the highest in the normoglycemic and lowest in the hyperglycemic subjects.

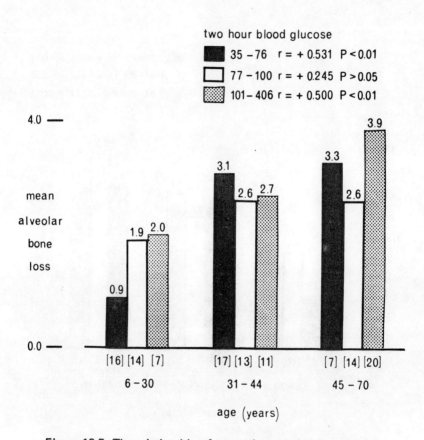

Figure 13-5. The relationship of age and mean alveolar bone loss in terms of two-hour (after loading) blood glucose. Statistically significant correlations exist only in the hyper- and hypoglycemic subjects and the highest correlation is noted in the low blood glucose group.

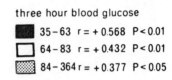

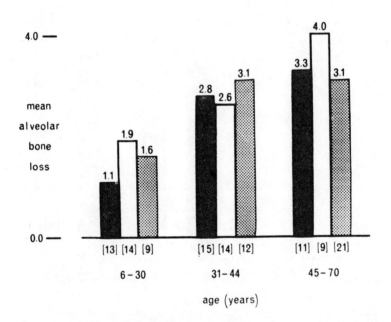

Figure 13-6. The relationship of age and mean alveolar bone loss in terms of three-hour (after loading) blood glucose. Statistically significant correlations exist in all three groups with the highest correlation in the hypoglycemic and lowest in the hyperglycemic subjects.

noteworthy that the two-hour post-load time is very comparable to the two-hour postprandial period which is recognized by many authorities as the best no-load point to measure glucose.[5]

Nontolerance Test

Claude Bernard, many years ago, pointed out that life and death are a function of homeostasis, meaning the steady state. He, and many others since then, have shown that the steady state is indeed most steady, meaning that health is characterized by small variations and disease is accompanied by wide fluctuations in clinical and biochemical parameters.[6-7]

Figure 13-7 pictorially portrays the concept of homeostasis. For example, a healthy individual's temperature fluctuates minimally during the day. In the ill the undulations are exaggerated. In the well the psychic state wavers slightly from minimal elation to marginal depression; in the sick, the manic-depressive cycles are abrupt and obvious. And so it is with blood pressure, peristalsis, and other clinical and biochemical parameters.

Figure 13-8 is simply an extension of figure 13-7 over a period of years. In the very early stages of chronic disease the amplitudes simply increase. With additional time, the broader undulations slowly begin to climb. Eventually, there is a leveling off characterized, for example, by hyperglycemia in diabetes mellitus and hypertension in heart disease.

From the description just offered, it follows that relatively young individuals (for example, under 40 years of age) in the main show relatively small variations in different clinical and biochemical areas. With advancing time, the amplitudes increase and slowly rise. This is pictorially indicated in figure 13-9. This biochemical pattern is consistent with the clinical course of events as shown in chapter 4.

To demonstrate this point, 272 presumably healthy

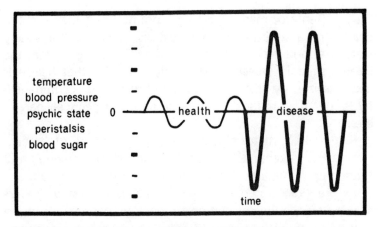

Figure 13-7. Health and disease can be plotted in a host of parameters. In health temperature, blood pressure, psychic state, peristalsis, blood sugar, et cetera, can be represented by small daily fluctuations. In disease the amplitudes are bigger.

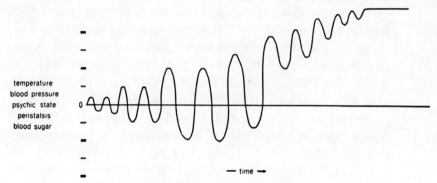

temperature
blood pressure
psychic state
peristalsis
blood sugar

— time —

Figure 13-8. An extension of Figure 7 over a period of years. In the early stages of chronic disease the amplitudes simply increase. With additional time the broader undulations slowly begin to climb. Eventually, there is a leveling off (e.g., hyperglycemia in diabetes mellitus, hypertension in heart disease, mania in certain psychiatric disorders).

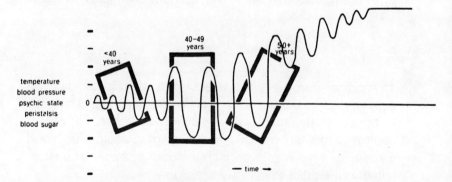

temperature
blood pressure
psychic state
peristalsis
blood sugar

— time —

Figure 13-9. A reexamination of Figure 13-8 showing that, with age, the amplitudes become larger and the mean scores slowly climb.

individuals were studied in terms of blood glucose at 8:30 a.m., 10:30 a.m., 12:30 p.m., 2:30 p.m., and 4:30 p.m. under *usual* conditions, meaning *without* any loading.[2] Figure 13-10 shows the means and standard deviations for these diurnal blood glucose patterns in the relatively young (less than 40 years), in the intermediate group (40-49 years), and in the elderly subjects (50+ years). Figure 13-10 shows that with advancing time the mean scores slowly rise. Also demonstrated is a slow but inevitable increase in variance. Hence, here is a quantitative demonstration of the patterns described earlier (figure 13-8 and 13-9).

Finally, figure 13-11 is intended to show the difference in diurnal blood glucose in elderly subjects (50+ years) who are relatively well (as judged by few clinical symptoms and signs) and relatively sick (as measured by many clinical symptoms and signs). Two points are clearly demonstrated. First, the mean fluctuations are greater in the ill (on the right) than in the well (on the left). Second, the overall fluctuations as judged by variances are decidedly larger in the sick group. This, again, confirms the story described in figures 13-8 and 13-9.

Summary

The prime purpose with tolerance testing is to elicit an exaggerated response to a particular stimulus. This, for instance, is the intent when glucose loading is utilized to determine the glucose tolerance pattern. Steroid plus blood glucose loading is an even more obvious example of a stress stimulus intended to magnify a response.

In a predictive medicine system the hope is to ascertain predisposition or early evidence of pathosis. To accomplish this end, data obtained under usual or routine (not stressed) circumstances serve adequately if it is recognized that physiologic and normal values are not synonymous and that subtle changes may be predictive.

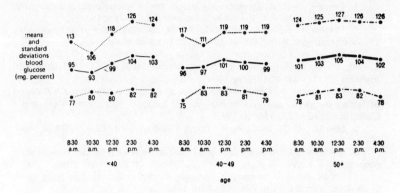

Figure 13-10. Means and standard deviations for diurnal blood glucose (without loading) in different age groups. There is evidence that the mean values slowly climb and the variances (amplitudes) slowly increase.

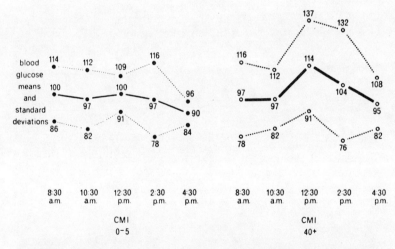

Figure 13-11. Mean and standard deviations for diurnal blood glucose (without loading) in subjects 50+ years old with relatively few general symptoms and signs (CMI 0-5) and many (CMI 40+). In the relatively sick group, the mean values are more variable and the variances (amplitudes) distinctly greater.

149

Predictive Medicine

References

1. Schoen, A. W. *Automated multiphasic health testing programs directory,* 1971-1972, second edition. Burbank, Bioscience Publications, Inc.

2. Cheraskin, E. and Ringsdorf, W. M., Jr. *Predictive medicine: XIII. Tolerance testing.* J. Amer. Geriat. Soc. 20:3, 121-126, March 1972.

3. Cheraskin, E., Ringsdorf, W. M., Jr., Setyaadmadja, A. T. S. H., and Barrett, R. A. *Clinical chemistry and predictive medicine.* J. Med. Assn. St. Alabama 36:11, 1337-1340, May 1967.

4. Fretham, A. A. *Clinics on endocrine and metabolic diseases. 10. Relation of fasting blood glucose level to oral glucose tolerance curve.* Staff Meet. Mayo Clinic 38:6, 110-115, 13 March 1963.

5. Shuman, C. R. *Diabetes detection.* Postgrad. Med. 45:4, 129-132, April 1969.

6. Sollberger, A. *How are biological time series related to the normal values concept?* Ann. New York Acad. Sc. 161:2, 606-625, 30 September 1969.

7. Shock, N. W. *Homeostatic disturbances and adaptations in aging.* Bull. Swiss Acad. Med. Sc. 24:4, 284-298, April 1968.

Results

When your work speaks for itself, don't interrupt.   —Henry J. Kaiser.

The purpose of the first thirteen chapters was to establish concepts and set the stage for an operational predictive medicine program. Broadly speaking, prediction is possible when two variables significantly coexist. For prognostic purposes, one factor need not be the cause of the other. In the earlier chapters, many such relationships were recounted. However, it is helpful when there is *also* cause-and-effect, for only then can one effect change in one variable by altering the other.

The purposes of this chapter are twofold.[1] First, to illustrate the changes (such as slowing, stopping, or reversing pathosis) which are possible during the early, amorphous incubation period of chronic disease. Second, by so doing, to resolve the oft-repeated question regarding the *effectiveness* of multiple testing programs. Many investigators[2-7] have rightly pointed out that there is a paucity of data to demonstrate that the course of disease is significantly altered as a result of multiphasic testing programs.

Therapeutic Techniques

A coronary thrombosis or the passing of a kidney stone are associated with severe pain. Therefore they require potent medication (e.g., morphine). But, under much less serious circumstances several million people in this country take sedatives, analgesics, and hypnotics on a regular basis. If one starts with the assumption that the *real* indication for an aspirin, for example, is an aspirin deficiency, then it follows that very few truly therapeutic tools are available.

In practical terms, the need is to add *resistance* agents and

14

151

so discourage the onset of chronic disease and to minimize *susceptibility* factors which favor the development of pathosis (chapter 3). In this perspective, diet (chapter 9) and physical activity (chapter 10) represent the simplest and most practical therapeutic armamentaria.

For these reasons, this chapter will consider the changes in clinical state, performance, biochemical status, and enzyme levels which are possible by modifying the diet[8] and altering physical activity.

Early Cardiovascular Symptoms and Signs

Mention was made in chapter 11 that man may be viewed as a lamellated sphere. The most peripheral layers represent the clinical state as judged by symptoms and signs. The point has also been made (chapter 4) that chronic disease commences with a few isolated findings which, with time, increase until a classical diagnosis is possible.

To demonstrate the effect of diet upon the clinical state, 171 dental practitioners and 128 wives were studied in terms of reported daily vitamin E consumption and reported cardiovascular symptoms and signs.[9] From this group, a second clinical-dietary comparison was made on 58 males and 37 females approximately one year later. Four items warrant special mention. First, the data confirm the well-established clinical fact that, with advancing age, there is an increase in the frequency of cardiovascular findings (figure 14-1). Second, an examination of the relationship between age and reported cardiovascular findings in both the males (figure 14-2) and females (figure 14-3) shows that the increase in clinical findings parallels age *only* in the subjects consuming less than the Recommended Dietary Allowance (RDA) for vitamin E. Additionally, the difference in the number of cardiovascular symptoms and signs is most sharply evident in the relatively oldest subjects. Finally, a review of the clinical change during the experimental year reveals that the decrease in cardiovascular findings (group I) occurred only in the

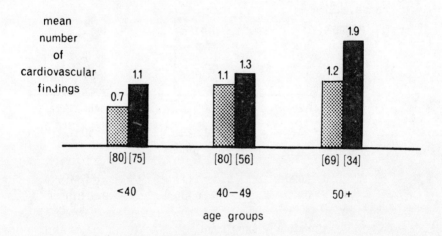

*statistically significant

Figure 14-1. The relationship of age (on the abscissa) and the frequency of reported cardiovascular findings (on the ordinate). In both the male and female groups, there is a low but statistically significant correlation.

153

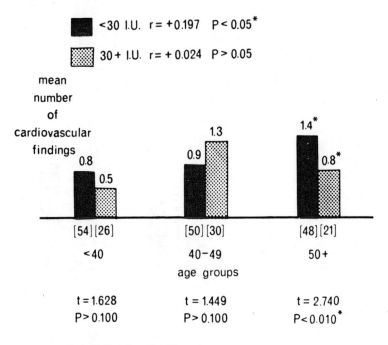

*statistically significant

Figure 14-2. The relationship of age (on the x-axis) and reported cardiovascular findings (on the y-axis) in terms of reported daily vitamin E intake <30 I.U. (black columns) and 30+ I.U. (stippled bars) in male subjects. With advancing age, there is a statistically significant (r = +0.197, P <0.05) increase in cardiovascular symptoms and signs only in the group consuming less than 30 I.U. daily which is below the Recommended Dietary Allowances. Additionally, intragroup examination by age shows only a statistically significant difference (t = 2.740, P <0.01) in the oldest age category (50+ years).

θ

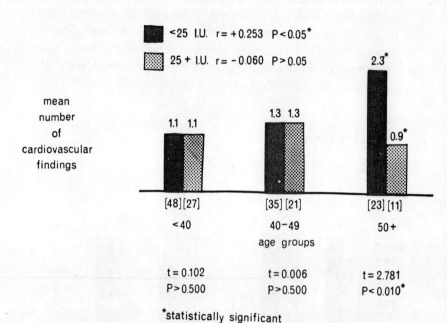

Figure 14-3. The relationship of age (on the abscissa) and reported cardiovascular findings (on the ordinate) in terms of reported daily vitamin E intake <25 I.U. (black columns) and 25+ I.U. (stippled bars) in female subjects. With advancing age there is a statistically significant (r = +0.253, P <0.05) increase in cardiovascular symptoms and signs only in the group consuming less that 25 I.U. daily, which is below the Recommended Dietary Allowances. Additionally, intragroup examination by age shows only a statistically significant difference (t = 2.781, P <0.01) in the oldest age category (50+ years).

155

group of subjects characterized by an increase in daily vitamin E intake (figure 14-4).

It is significant that early cardiovascular findings can be reduced or eliminated *before* the onset of classical heart disease. It is also noteworthy that this clinical reversal can be accomplished by relatively simple dietary techniques. Most importantly, this example demonstrates the effectiveness of a predictive medicine multiple testing program.

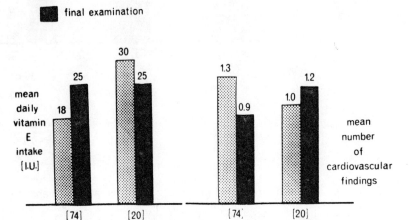

*statistically significant

Figure 14-4. The relationship of change in reported daily vitamin E intake (left side) and change in reported cardiovascular symptoms and signs (right side) in subjects who increased daily vitamin E intake (group I) and who decreased daily vitamin E (group III). Only in group I is there a reduction (1.3 to 0.9 complaints per person) in cardiovascular findings of statistical import (t = 2.602, P <0.025).

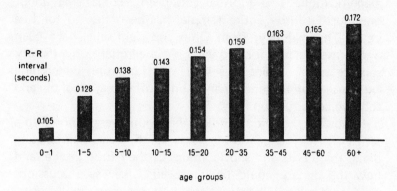

Figure 14-5. The relationship of the P-R interval (in seconds) to age in 872 normal persons. It is clear that, with time, the P-R interval lengthens.

Early Electrocardiographic Evidence of Disease

It is generally held that, with advancing age, the P-R interval lengthens.[10-11] Figure 14-5 pictorially portrays the duration of $P-R_1$ in different age groups. The question arises as to whether this particular characteristic of the aging process can be regarded as *normal* or *physiologic.* Parenthetic mention should be made that this topic has been earlier reviewed (chapter 6). On the assumption that normal is synonymous with average, it is clear that, with age, it is indeed normal for the P-R interval to lengthen. However, it is possible to demonstrate that it is not physiologic to show a progressively longer P-R interval with time.

Two hundred fifty dentists and their wives, participants in a multiple testing program in Florida under the auspices of the Southern Academy of Clinical Nutrition, in Los Angeles under the aegis of the Southern California Academy of Nutritional Research, and in Columbus under the sponsorship of the Ohio Academy of Clinical Nutrition, shared in this experiment.[12] A standard three-limb lead electrocardiogram was taken. The P-R interval was measured carefully under magnification. The Florida contingent, comprising about one-fourth of the entire sample, has been studied for five years. The majority, from Ohio and California, have been under investigation for two years. At the initial study, dietary surveys were obtained as well as information concerning exercise, vitamin supplementation, coffee/tea, alcohol, and tobacco consumption.

Following the initial studies, the groups were exposed to a series of health education lectures pointing out their existing diets, the merits and shortcomings of their food intake, and how the dietary could be improved. Likewise, discussions were held regarding physical activity, vitamin supplementation, coffee/tea, alcohol, and tobacco consumption.

Electrocardiograms, dietary surveys, and records of physical activity, et cetera, were repeated almost annually providing an opportunity to ascertain the electrocardiographic changes in the light of diet, exercise, et cetera.

Figure 14-6 shows by stippled bars the norms previously described (figure 14-5). Superimposed (black columns) are the initial findings for the group of seemingly healthy dentists and their wives. Two points are evident. First, in the dental group there is a lengthening of the P-R interval with time. Second, the mean value at each temporal point is lower for the dentists and their wives than it is for the Lepeschkin sample.

Following the initial observations, the dietary habits of the group were discussed. It was found that, generally speaking, the refined carbohydrate intake was high, the protein consumption low, and the vitamin-mineral intake suboptimal when compared with the Recommended Dietary Allowances outlined by the Food and Nutrition Board of the National Research Council. Additionally, it was learned that a significant number of individuals reported no daily physical activity. These defects were pointed out to the group and discussions were held as to how to improve the dietary and to introduce an exercise program. Subsequently, dietary surveys

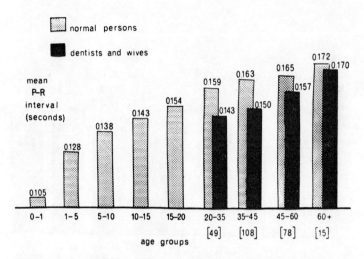

Figure 14-6. The relationship of age and the P-R interval in normal persons (stippled columns) versus the findings in presumably healthy dentists and their wives (black columns). In both groups, the P-R interval lengthens with time. However, the rate is much slower in the professional group.

demonstrated that a notable segment of the group had altered food intake significantly, as judged by less refined carbohydrate food substances, greater quantities of protein, and more vitamins and minerals. Additionally, the data revealed that a large number of the group had inaugurated some form of daily exercise.

Figure 14-7 shows the baseline data of Lepeschkin by means of the light (stippled) bars. Superimposed are cross-hatched columns showing the mean P-R interval values at the start of the experimental period and black bars for the mean P-R intervals following the health education lecture series. Two items should be underlined. First, with time, the P-R interval lengthens in each category. Second, at each temporal

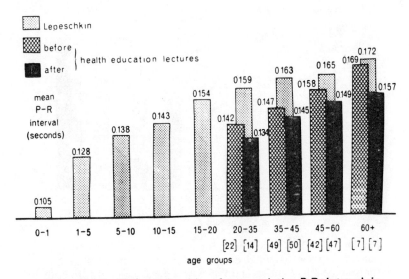

Figure 14-7. The relationship of age and the P-R interval in normal persons (lightly stippled columns) and in the dentists and their wives before (hatched bars) and after health education lectures (black columns).

point, the mean P-R interval is less after health education lectures than before.

The evidence here demonstrates that the initial P-R intervals in these dentists and their wives are better (shorter) than in the established norms. This is very likely due to the fact, as has been pointed out elsewhere,[13] that it is the health-conscious dentist who tends to participate in a health evaluation program. Finally, the data shown here suggest that the P-R interval may be shortened following health education lectures. This is graphically portrayed in figure 14-8. Line a-a shows that the oldest group of subjects (60+ years) after health education lectures showed a mean P-R interval of 0.157 seconds. Line a-a shows that this is less than the P-R interval (0.158 seconds) prior to health education instruction for the 45-60 year age group. A similar reversal is pictured (line b-b) at ages 35-45 versus 20-35. Actually, in every age group, the P-R interval after health education lectures was reduced to that found in persons 15-20 years younger.

It is recognized that health and disease are multifactorial problems in a study of this type. It is impossible to develop strict control. Thus, it must be appreciated that the changes in the P-R interval are very likely due to a *combination* of changes in the habits of the group. However, for purposes of this discussion, physical activity will also be considered independently.

Figure 14-9 shows four groups: (1) those who carried out daily exercise at the start and through to the end of the experimental period, (2) those who instituted exercise following the initial studies, (3) those who discontinued exercise during the experimental period, and (4) those who engaged in no physical activity during the entire period. It will be observed (figure 14-9) that the only statistically significant reduction (t = 2.897, P <0.01) in the P-R interval occurred in the group who instituted physical activity during the survey period. Hence, this circumstantial evidence, in line with other data,[14] underlines the possible cause-and-effect relationship of physical activity to one electrocardiographic parameter.

Summary

Much has been written about the nature and causes of the aging process. For purposes of a predictive medicine program, four points serve as a reasonable base. First, old people report more symptoms and signs. Second, old people die more readily than young people. Third, old people with many clinical findings die more readily than old people with few

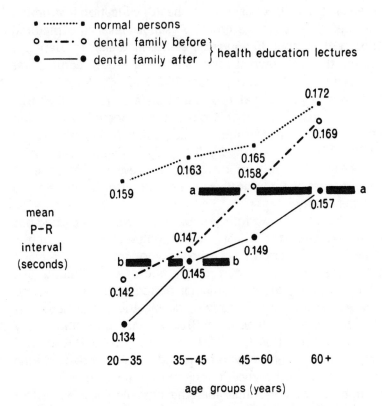

Figure 14-8. Lines a-a and b-b show that, following health education lectures, the mean P-R interval shortens, suggesting that, as the group becomes chronologically older, it becomes electrocardiographically younger.

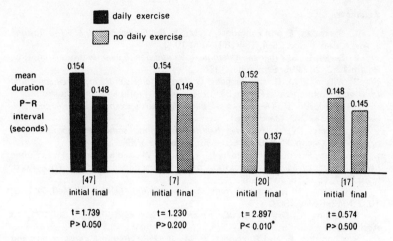

Figure 14-9. The relationship of a change in physical activity and a change in P-R$_1$ duration during a one-year period. No significant change occurred in the groups characterized by daily exercise at the start and end of the year, no daily exercise during the experiment, or in those who stopped daily physical activity. There was a statistically significant reduction in the P-R interval only in the group that started to exercise following the initial study.

symptoms and signs. Therefore it follows that it is highly desirable to utilize all techniques possible to reduce the number of clinical findings to a minimum. Needless to say, the medical facilities required to care for people so treated would be less than in traditional medical systems.

Examples are offered here to show that this is possible. By so doing, it becomes clear that a predictive medicine program can indeed be successful in the anticipation of classical textbook disease. One instance is cited to show that the supposed inevitable increase of cardiovascular symptoms and signs can be thwarted by dietary means (vitamin E). A second example is offered to demonstrate that, in part by exercise and/or diet, people can be made younger at heart!

Predictive Medicine

References

1. Cheraskin, E. and Ringsdorf, W. M., Jr. *Predictive medicine: XIV. Results.* J. Amer. Geriat. Soc. 20:4, 184-189, April 1972.
2. Siegel, G. S. *American dilemma—periodic health examination.* Arch. Env. Health 13:3, 292-295, September 1966.
3. Wilson, J. M. G. and Jungner, G. *The principles and practice of screening for disease.* Public Health Papers 34, 1968. Geneva, World Health Organization.
4. David, W. D. *Usefulness of periodic health examinations.* Arch. Env. Health 2:3, 339-342, March 1961.
5. Roberts, N. J. *Periodic health evaluation: some developments and practices.* J. Occup. Med. 8:11, 581-588, November 1966.
6. Kruse, H. D., Baumgartner, L., Kolbe, H. W., and McCarthy, H. L. *Public health aspects of aging: transcription of panel meeting.* Bull. New York Acad. Med. 33:7, 493-518, July 1957.
7. Thorner, R. M. *Whither multiphasic screening?* New Eng. J. Med. 280:19, 1037-1042, 8 May 1969.
8. Pauling, L. *Orthomolecular psychiatry.* Science 160:3825, 265-271, 19 April 1968.
9. Cheraskin, E. and Ringsdorf, W. M., Jr. *Daily vitamin E consumption and reported cardiovascular findings.* Nutr. Rep. Internat. 2:2, 107-117, August 1970.
10. Lepeschkin, E. *Modern electrocardiography.* 1951. Baltimore, The Williams and Wilkens Company. p. 153.
11. Simonson, E. *Differentiation between normal and abnormal in electrocardiography.* 1961. Saint Louis, The C. V. Mosby Company.
12. Cheraskin, E. and Ringsdorf, W. M., Jr. *Younger at heart: a study of the P-R interval.* J. Amer. Geriat. Soc. 19:3, 271-275, March 1971.
13. Editorial. *ADA Health Screening Program.* J. A. D. A. 79:2, 235-236, August 1969.
14. Cureton, T. K. *The physiological effects of exercise programs on adults.* 1969. Springfield, Charles C. Thomas. pp. 64, 78, 84.

Epilogue

Plans are the dreams of the reasonable. —Feuchtersleben.

According to the latest available figures (1967) cited by the United States Department of Health, Education, and Welfare,[1] approximately three and one-half million persons are presently engaged in occupations related to health services (figure 15-1). This is in sharp contrast to two and one-half million just seven years previously and tenfold greater than the manpower source at the turn of the century. According to the same source, the figure will rise to well over five million in a decade *if health care is simply to be maintained at the present level.*

In the year 1929[2-3] the United States spent three and one-half billion dollars for all medical care. This means, in the light of the one hundred million Americans living at that time, that the average cost per person per year was thirty-five dollars, or less than ten cents a day (figure 15-2). In 1967-1968 the nation spent fifty billion dollars for two hundred million people. This is two hundred fifty dollars per person per annum, or sixty-eight cents daily for every man, woman, and child. For 1970[4] the cost of medical care reached sixty-one billion dollars. This is five times the 1950 price and fifteenfold that of 1930. In 1971 the health care bill was a staggering 79 billion dollars. Health care services in 1972 are expected to total almost 88 billion dollars. Spending for health care is expected to rise at an annual rate of 8.5 percent throughout the seventies, reaching more than 113 billion dollars by 1975 and almost 169 billion by 1980.

There is a second way to view the health economics problem. This is possible by analyzing the percentage of the national effort (the gross national product) which is utilized for medical care. In 1929 medical expenditures usurped 3.6

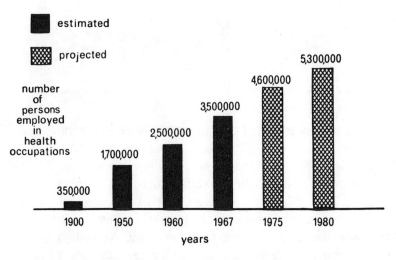

Figure 15-1. The estimated number of persons employed in health occupations, and the projections to 1980 (stippled columns).

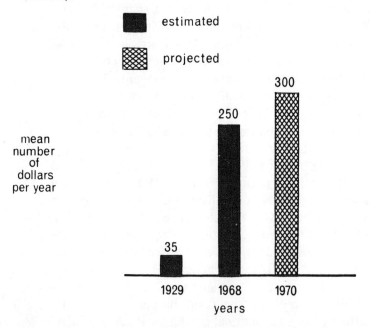

Figure 15-2. Estimated (black columns) and projected (stippled columns) dollar cost per year per capita for health care.

cents out of every dollar earned. In 1968-1969, the figure had ballooned to 6 cents. The most up-to-date figure (1972) is that 8 percent of the gross national product will be swallowed up for medical purposes.

There is still a third way to assess the problem. In 1929 taxes paid for 13 percent of medical costs in the United States. Today it is 40 percent. Hence, there has been a greater than threefold increase.

Fourth, there are significant hospital figures.[1-4] In 1965 hospital costs were rising at the rate of 8 to 9 percent per year. This was twice as fast as the rise in the cost of living. In 1963 hospital costs were projected to double in eight years. For example, hospitals like the Cornell Medical Center were charging about 60 dollars per day. It was, therefore, estimated that in eight years (1971) the daily costs would climb to 120 dollars. Actually, the projections were quite accurate. For instance, many hospitals today charge 100 dollars per day. The compounded rate of increase in 1968 was 15 percent. If this trend continues, it means that hospital costs will double again, this time in five instead of eight years. Thus, daily hospital rates should be 200 dollars a day in 1973 and 400 dollars daily in 1978. At that time a six-week heart attack will cost, for hospital care alone, almost 17,000 dollars. According to American Medical News,[5] *hospital costs in the major urban areas could reach 1,000 dollars per day within ten years.*

With these manpower and financial figures as background,[6] it is well to examine the health status in the United States. Broadly speaking, the efforts should extend in three directions. First, diagnosis and treatment of disease on a one-to-one basis. Second, the large and highly organized multiple testing programs. Third, the application of predictive concepts.

The health of a society has been traditionally measured by the rate at which its members draw their last breaths. Hence, the simplest data are *mortality* figures.

167

In recent times the concept has undergone considerable modification. There is new interest in the total quality of life and not just the life-span. Thus, *morbidity* statistics are receiving more attention. In other words, data are available to show the incidence and prevalence of many diseases such as cancer, diabetes mellitus, heart disease, and blindness.

There is very limited information to indicate how many people are just ailing with nonspecific complaints like insomnia, diarrhea, headaches, and nervousness. These people have not yet developed enough complaints for the findings to fit a precise category. This is required in traditional medical diagnosis before the disease can be labeled with such terms as cancer, heart disease, or schizophrenia.

Even among allegedly healthy subjects there are over two hundred so-called multiple testing health evaluation programs in operation designed to ascertain early illness.[7] However, as far as the evaluation of disease proneness is concerned, there are only very meager efforts devoted to true predictive systems.

Death Rates

It is alarming but true that, concerning infant mortality ranked by country, the United States is eighteenth with 24.8 deaths per 1,000 live births. For life expectancy at birth among the same nations the United States is twenty-first with 66.6 years. The Netherlands heads the list with 71.4 years. Thus, though the American gross national product is much greater, the Dutch have a life expectancy at birth of almost five years more.[8]

With all the billions that have been spent for health care in the United States since 1900, the 45-year-old white male has gained only three years in life expectancy. Above this age the increase quickly dwindles to insignificance. For example, the 60-year-old white male can expect to live only one and one-half years longer than his grandfather did.

The evidence from mortality figures suggests that the present approach to health care leaves much to be desired.[9]

Classical Morbidity Figures

According to recent releases by the United States National Center for Health Statistics, killing and crippling diseases are alarmingly prevalent.[10] For example, 13.2 percent of Americans in the 45-54-year-age group have heart disease. By the time the general population reaches 75+ years, almost one person of every two has a cardiac problem. Another revealing fact comes from a recent report by the American Heart Association[11] which states that, for adults 20 years of age and older, 27,000,000 Americans are living with some form of cardiovascular pathosis. This means that one out of every eight Americans suffers with cardiovascular disease.

The United States National Center for Health Statistics[10] also notes that approximately one out of ten Americans at the age of 45-54 has arthritis-rheumatism. This figure climbs above one in four in the age group of 75+. Figures are also available for diabetes mellitus (ranging as high as 3 to 4 percent), asthma (about 5 percent), hearing deficits (26 percent), and visual impairment (17 percent).

The obvious point of these figures is that the present health-care methods are not adequate to resolve the *morbidity* patterns of the nation.

The Nonspecific Ailing Group

Chronic disorders generally develop over an extended period of time. It is a fact that one does not retire well and awaken the following morning with a chronic disease. Thus, the classical identification of these problems is preceded by an incubation period, in some cases of many years duration (chapter 4). It is during this time that the patient begins to notice the appearance of various symptoms and signs. Many findings are nonspecific, such as insomnia, fatigue, nervousness, and anorexia.

Quantitative information regarding the incidence and prevalence of this type of information is very limited. One interesting source comes from observations of members of the health professions (physicians and dentists).

A multiple testing program was conducted at an annual convention of the American Medical Association.[12] The program was very superficial and included a short questionnaire, a limited battery of biochemical tests, and an electrocardiogram. The evidence derived indicated that about one in three physicians tested had an elevated serum cholesterol level, one in five had hyperglycemia, and about one in three showed hyperuricemia. These sparse figures are noteworthy for several reasons. First, it should be pointed out that it is usually the relatively young and healthy physicians who participate in these health projects. Thus, the figures for physicians overall would likely be higher. Second, the testing program was very restricted. It is likely that, if more parameters were studied, more problems would be discovered.

It would appear, from these bits of evidence, that the existing health system is not satisfying the needs of the millions of people with early and nonspecific symptoms and signs.

Health Evaluation Programs

It must be admitted that it is difficult to differentiate between those with illnesses in the early incubation period and those with good health. One of the difficulties lies in the fact that no one is *perfectly* healthy. Fortunately, increasing attention is being given to the study of *presumably* healthy persons. These ongoing multitesting programs run the gamut from executive personnel in Philadelphia to longshoremen in San Francisco.[13] The incidence of *previously* unrecognized *significant* disease varies widely depending upon the age sample, socioeconomic status, health awareness, and the scope of the testing techniques. However, the data show quite clearly that somewhere between 65 and 95 percent of presumably *healthy* people are *not* healthy.[14] This should come as no surprise when it is realized that 95 percent of Americans suffer with dental caries and/or periodontal pathosis, which clearly are not signs of health.

Hence, at this level, there is considerable progress. The multiple testing concept has developed a high degree of data collection with the use of computers and automated data systems. It has demonstrated that mass analysis can be accomplished at a reasonable cost. It has brought into focus the fact that, even among the so-called healthy, there is a large reservoir of disease. However, these massive data collection systems have not accomplished a change in the mortality and morbidity trends of the nation. The reason for this failure is that these multiphasic screening *health* programs are *not* health programs. In fact, they are highly organized and beautifully executed *disease detection* systems.[15]

Predictive Systems

A true health program must have, as its fundamental thesis, the anticipation and prevention rather than the identification and treatment of disease (chapter 1). At the present time no such formal program exists anywhere in the world. *As a matter of fact, the whole intent of this monograph is to describe the gross anatomy of such a system.*

There are isolated individuals and centers concerned with areas which rightfully fit into a predictive medicine program. For example, Stamler and his colleagues have attained a high prognostic level with regard to coronary artery disease.[16]

An ongoing survey of 433 dentists and their wives currently operational in Los Angeles under the auspices of the Southern California Academy of Nutritional Research, in Columbus under the direction of the Ohio Academy of Clinical Nutrition, and in Florida under the sponsorship of the Southern Academy of Clinical Nutrition is perhaps the best model of a predictive medicine program.

The program is unique because it appreciates the thesis of

anticipating rather than identifying disease (chapter 1). The project is singular by virtue of its sensitivity to proneness profiles (chapter 2). The survey operates from a base designed to identify factors which contribute to host resistance and susceptibility (chapter 3). There is a built-in recognition of the gradation of disease from an early nonspecific pattern of seemingly diverse and independent symptoms and signs to the eventual culmination of the clinical course with a distinct diagnostic label (chapter 4). Perhaps one of the most critical ingredients is an awareness that *peripheral* health and disease, as judged by clinical symptoms and signs, are parabolically related to biochemical state (chapter 5). Additionally, the predictive implications have been enhanced by the thesis that the so-called normal ranges are not synonymous with physiologic values (chapter 6). The program is further unique because it is cognizant that testing parameters, while they may be characteristic of a syndrome, are not pathognomonic (chapter 7). It becomes abundantly clear from a study of the membership of this survey that environmental influences play a more significant role in the genesis of disease than heretofore held (chapter 8). Finally, this program places great emphasis on diet (chapter 9), exercise (chapter 10), and the oral cavity (chapter 11). All of the survey information has been collected under natural conditions so that a picture can be developed of the individual as he actually is in his own environment (chapter 13).

The results of the program are exciting and a departure from anything reported by the traditional medical method (chapter 14). For example, the subjects who showed an increase in daily vitamin E consumption also demonstrated a decrease in reported cardiovascular symptoms and signs. The individuals who began daily exercise displayed a decrease in the duration of the P-R interval in Lead I. There was a significant reduction in nonfasting serum cholesterol and serum triglycerides.[17]

On the other hand, there are a number of serious limitations in this embryonal predictive medicine program. First, the subjects are strewn across the country. In other words, there is no one locus to allow strict supervision of the data collection. Second, since the total cost is borne by the membership, the parameters which have been chosen are a function of economics. Finally, the anatomy of the program does not lend itself to built-in controls.

Summary

The fifteen chapters in this book are designed to outline the *strategy* of a predictive medicine program. Clearly, the *tactics* require additional investigation.

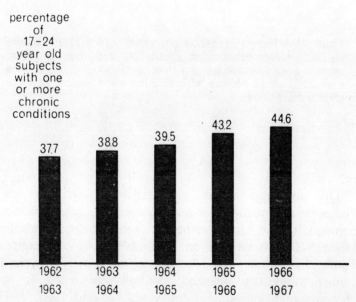

United States Department of Health. Education and Welfare, National Center for Health Statistics, Series 10. Numbers 5. 13. 25. 37 and 43. January 1964– January 1968. Current Estimates from the Health Interview Survey. Superintendent of Documents. United States Government Printing Office. Washington, D.C.

Figure 15-3. The percentage of the 17-24-year-old civilian, noninstitutionalized population with one or more chronic conditions during the years 1962 to 1967.

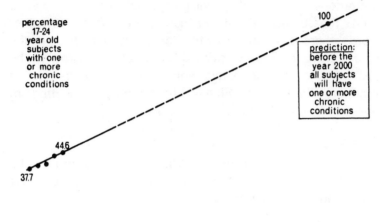

Figure 15-4. Projections showing the trend in the 17-24-year-old civilian, noninstitutionalized population with one or more chronic conditions. According to these extrapolations, by the year 2000 all 17-24-year-old individuals will have one or more chronic conditions.

The justifications for a predictive system are many. Perhaps the best reason is that conventional medicine is not coping with and cannot manage the existing disease problem. Much has been written on this subject. As one example, figure 15-3 shows the percentage of the 17-24-year-old civilian, noninstitutionalized population with one or more chronic conditions during the years 1962 to 1967.[18] The figures are significant because of the high incidence in 1962 (37.7 percent) and the steady climb to 44.6 percent in 1967. What is more disturbing are the projections (figure 15-4).

174

According to the best available information, at the present rate, *all* 17-24-year-old subjects will be afflicted before the turn of the century!

However, there is a remedy—*predictive medicine!*

References

1. Pennell, M. Y. and Hoover, D. B. *Health manpower source book 21: allied health manpower supply and requirements: 1950-80.* United States Department of Health, Education, and Welfare. Public Health Service Publication 263, Section 21. 1970. Washington, D. C., United States Government Printing Office.

2. Ubell, E. *Too much too late (a speech to the Caduceus Society of Cornell Medical College).* Prevention 21:9, 57-68, September 1969.

3. Jones, B. *The health of Americans.* 1970. Englewood Cliffs, New Jersey, Prentice-Hall, Inc.

4. U. S. Department of Commerce. *U. S. Industrial outlook 1972 with projections to 1980.* Superintendant of documents, U. S. Government Printing Office, Washington, D. C. 1972.

5. Medicine's Week. *$1,000-a-day hospital rooms seen.* Amer. Med. News, p. 2, 4 May 1970.

6. Ginzberg. E. *Men, money, and medicine.* 1969. New York, Columbia University Press.

7. Schoen, A. W. *Automated multiphasic health testing programs directory,* 1971-1972, second edition. Burbank, Bioscience Publications, Inc.

8. United Nations Demographic Yearbook, 1964 and 1965.

9. Schuman, L. M. *Approaches to primary prevention of disease.* Pub. Health Rep. 85:1, 1-10, January 1970.

10. Twaddle, A. C. *Aging, population growth and chronic illness.* J. Chron. Dis. 21:6, 417-422, October 1968.

11. American Heart Association, 44 East 23rd Street, New York, New York. *Heart facts.* PR-33, 1970.

12. Editorial. *You may be sicker than you think.* J. A. M. A. 181:12, 27, 22 September 1962.

13. Roberts, N. J. *Periodic health maintenance examinations.* In Hubbard, J. P. *The early detection and prevention of disease.* 1957. New York, The Blakiston Division, McGraw-Hill Book Company. pp. 27-57.

14. Schenthal, J. E. *Multiphasic screening of the well patient: twelve year experience of the Tulane University Cancer Detection Clinic.* J. A. M. A. 172:1, 51-54, 2 January 1960.

15. Symposium. *Automated multiphasic health testing in the seventies.* Westchester County Medical Society, 14 January 1970.

16. Stamler, J. *Lectures on preventive cardiology.* 1967. New York, Grune and Stratton, Inc.

17. Cheraskin, E. and Ringsdorf, W. M., Jr. *Predictive medicine: XV. Epilogue.* J. Amer. Geriat. Soc. 20:6, pp. 279-283, June 1972.

18. National Center for Health Statistics. *Current estimates from The Health Interview Survey.* Series 10:5, 13, 25, 37, 43, January 1964-January 1968. Washington, D. C., United States Government Printing Office.

GENERAL INDEX

178

INDEX TO FIGURES AND TABLES